Y0-CQB-881

3 0000 002 392 755

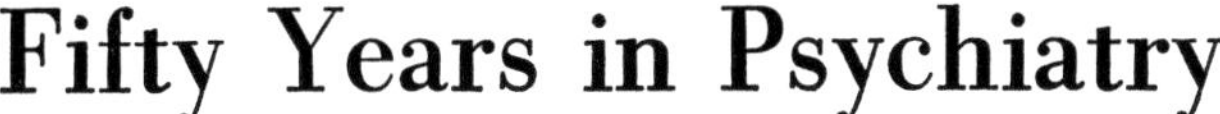
Fifty Years in Psychiatry

FIFTY YEARS IN PSYCHIATRY

A Living History

By

ROY R. GRINKER, SR., M.D.

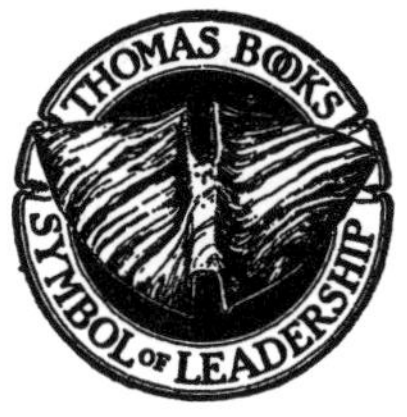

CHARLES C THOMAS · PUBLISHER
Springfield · Illinois · U.S.A.

Published and Distributed Throughout the World by

CHARLES C THOMAS • PUBLISHER

BANNERSTONE HOUSE

301-327 East Lawrence Avenue, Springfield, Illinois, U.S.A.

ISBN 0-398-03876-7

Library of Congress Catalog Card Number: 78-24355

With THOMAS BOOKS *careful attention is given to all details of manufacturing and design. It is the Publisher's desire to present books that are satisfactory as to their physical qualities and artistic possibilities and appropriate for their particular use.* THOMAS BOOKS *will be true to those laws of quality that assure a good name and good will.*

Printed in the United States of America

N-1

Library of Congress Cataloging in Publication Data

Grinker, Roy Richard, 1900-
Fifty years in psychiatry.

Bibliography: p. 242
Includes index.
1. Psychiatry—History. I. Title. [DNLM: 1. Psychiatry—History. 2. Psychiatry—Trends. WM11.1 G867f]
RC438.G74 616.8'9'0904 78-24355
ISBN 0-398-03876-7

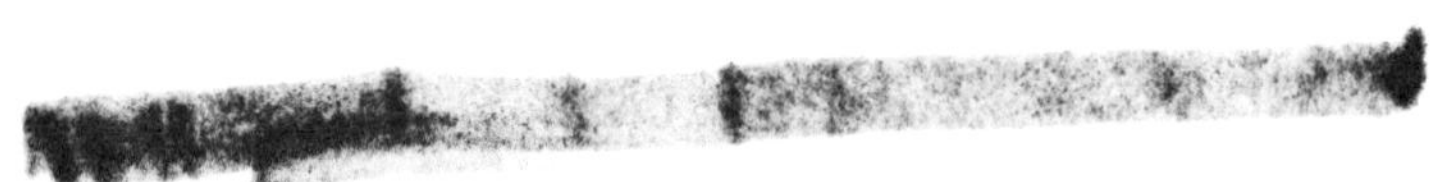

to

My Beloved Family

Mildred, Roy, Jr., M.D., Florence, Jennifer and Roy III

Preface

SCIENTIFIC and medical histories are difficult to write in the present, because so many authors and editors have articulated contradictory and conflicting points of view about the past. Every man has his own observations and biases, formed over the time span of his own life.

As Zilboorg (1943) has stated, when a physician writes for a general audience, he must mind his language and tell what is wrong, unmasking prejudices and false beliefs. In a sense, his role is a negative one—often overdone, to be sure, as such recent books as Szasz's *Myth of Mental Illness* (1961) and Torrey's *Death of Psychiatry* (1974) testify.

The potentially and acutely mentally ill are now considered as consumers; not only with the right to receive the best of care, but with the power to organize in order to inspect and monitor the work of the professionals. Intelligent consumerism, however, is hard to come by. The wide variety of fads, sects, and encounter groups that have recently burgeoned have made the public, and even psychiatrists, increasingly perplexed and antagonistic.

As a general psychiatrist, I shall try to define not only for the professional but also for concerned lay people—consumers, if you will—psychiatry. Psychiatry is not only a specialty of medicine, oriented toward treatment by a wide variety of methods, as most lay persons think; it is also a scientific discipline. Perhaps, it is more accurate to say that it has two faces: It has both a medical or scientific model and a humanistic or subjective model. Yet, these two perspectives actually overlap and interact. Jerome D. Frank (1977) wrote that the religious-magical and the scientific faces of psychology are increasingly resembling each other. As long ago as 1900, Sir William Osler (as quoted by Dubos, 1976) wrote on "the faith that heals." Indeed, the faith and belief systems constituting the existential humanistic approach lie closely beneath the scientific mask. Until the era of psychoanalysis, from the time of antiquity, faith, sugestion, support, and direction have constituted the main methods of therapy for persons in trouble.

Psychiatry, as seen from a biological perspective, developed only very slowly from the time I received my medical degree in 1921 until at least the 1950s. In summary, progress has been pitifully frustrating and discouraging. In the early years of this century, physicians practiced psychiatry *and* neurology, as so-called neuropsychiatrists, according to the medical model—with a strong bias toward "constitutional" or so-called organic causations.

What did psychiatrists do in those years? In clinical work, they utilized the Kraepelinian classification for diagnosis. Neuroses were treated in private practice by psychotherapies embodying suggestion, support, persuasion, and direction, and with small doses of sodium bromide. Later, phenobarbital, which my father introduced into this country from one of his postgraduate trips to Europe, was added, although this drug was primarily effective in the treatment of epilepsy, until it was eventually superseded by Dilantin®. Group, family, and behavior modification therapies as well as psychoanalysis still lay in the future.

The psychoses were the subject of the most boring lectures in the medical curriculum—discouraging to students with any interest in psychiatry. Most psychotic patients were sent far from their families (who were presumed to be pathogenic) to private sanatoriums, usually for a lifetime. The poor were warehoused in state mental hospitals for lives of misery and early deaths. There, the few staff psychiatrists spent their time arguing about the diagnosis and prescribing hydrotherapy, sedation, or restraint. Psychiatrists had difficulty in understanding the importance of varying the doses of pharmacological agents for individual patients and relied instead on so-called standard dosage. Initially, drug therapy was inept because it took a long time before side-effects were understood and tests for tolerance were developed.

Many psychiatrists placed their patients on so-called rest cures modeled after the theories developed by Weir Mitchell (1894) after the American Civil War. These included bed rest and high-fat diets to replenish the supposedly deteriorated myelin sheaths. Some neuropsychiatrists hospitalized their patients in general hospitals, using the false diagnosis of suspected brain tumor, because there were no available psychiatric units. Other patients were placed in hotels with nurses around the clock.

My professional career in psychiatry has spanned more than five decades, a period in which modern psychiatry has developed, matured, and met many challenges. However, many more remain unsolved. This should be an appropriate moment to give a backward glance at psychiatric history and to look forward into a clouded but illuminated crystal ball.

Others as well as myself have made previous attempts to contribute to a history of psychiatry. Michael Shepherd (1977) wrote about Sir Aubrey Lewis; Kurt Eissler (1965) wrote polemics about critics of Freud; Percival Bailey (1965) published a critique, *Sigmund the Unserene;* and Ilza Vieth (1967) wrote on the history of hysteria. I have written about the psychoanalytic island that existed in Chicago in 1911 to 1912 (1963a), about Lasswell's early psychosomatic studies, and have prepared an as yet unpublished history of the Chicago Institute for Psychoanalysis. Alexander and Selesnick (1966) have written a severely criticized history of psychiatry. Bry and Rifkin (1964) seem to recognize the difficulty of keeping up with the literature by writing that book reviews effectively document professional ideas and provide significant professional critiques of the time.

As we know, history is not a "hard" science. There are many ways of writing histories, depending on tastes, the range of activities in which the writer himself has been involved, and his own personality and special biases. History, as Carl Becker (1935) wrote, is "the memory of things said and done. Historical facts do not speak for themselves. They need the perceiving mind to reveal their special meaning."

That there are risks in the historical enterprise is clear enough. As Graubard (1974) wrote, "While there is always the hazard of mistaking one's own experience, within one's own institution or local community, to be representative of a larger, national pattern, there is much to be said for exploiting the knowledge that is made available through such observation."

I shall describe psychiatry as I knew it—considering it critically through a discussion of several broad topical issues, though details may inevitably be lost in the attempt to generalize and abstract the essential patterns. The thread of my own life and career cannot, of course, be disentangled from the total fiber. In my Benjamin Rush lecture at the American Psychiatric Association in 1970, I said, "The history of psychiatry and psychology in their *search for meaning* of human mentation in the health-illness continuum corresponds with the history of social dynamics and change, and with the story of individuals as they struggle in *their* search for meaning."

ROY R. GRINKER, SR., M.D.

Acknowledgment

MANY OF THE quotations in this volume are from my own work, published and unpublished.

Appreciation must be expressed to the editors of the books and journals in which my writings have appeared. I am especially grateful to the *Archives of General Psychiatry*, for permission to publish excerpts from articles that I wrote for that journal while I was its chief editor, and to Dr. Frances Braceland, for permission to publish excerpts from papers published in the *American Journal of Psychiatry*.

I am indebted to a number of co-authors of various papers. as well as to Philip Holzman, Martin Harrow, Doris Gruenewald, Mary Rootes, Don Schwartz, Froma Walsh, Marion Levin, Judith Beck, and Nat Apter, members of the schizophrenic research team at the Psychiatric and Psychosomatic Institute at Michael Reese Hospital in Chicago, who assisted in rating and diagnosing an undifferentiated sample of 337 young hospitalized patients. The separation of the 186 schizophrenics from the 151 nonschizophrenics, and the classifications of the schizophrenics into several groups, contributed significantly to the research. Special thanks are due to Philip Holzman, Ph.D., for his help in developing the schizophrenic planning document, which came out of our 1969 to 1970 discussions.

Mrs. Helene Burson, Carol Kennedy, and Shirlee Morris Dwyer have been most helpful in preparing the transcriptions of the material for this manuscript, and I am appreciative of their dedication and competence.

To Janice J. Feldstein, I acknowledge my intense gratitude for her expert editorial services. It was she who eliminated repetitions, strengthened the structure of each chapter, and eliminated unnecessary autobiographical details, which will be available at another time.

ROY R. GRINKER, SR., M.D.
Michael Reese Hospital and Medical Center
Institute for Psychosomatic and Psychiatric
Research and Training (P & PI)
Chicago, Illinois 60616

CONTENTS

Fifty Years in Psychiatry

CHAPTER 1

Introduction

My career in psychiatry was the result of several fortuitous circumstances. Through several accidental meetings, I was invited by Dean Franklin McLean to move away from Michael Reese Hospital, where I was working as a neurologist, to the University of Chicago, where I would replace an imported medical neurologist who had proved unsatisfactory. In 1929 I did so. The sections of neurology and neurosurgery (under Percival Bailey) were fused at the time, and all laboratories and resources were combined. We worked together to establish a unified training program.

Any physician specializing in neurology could take three years of residency; if he wanted to go into neurosurgery, he took one year of medical neurology and then went on to neurosurgery. Paul Bucy, Earl Walker, the professor of neurological surgery at Johns Hopkins, and Paul Levine at Texas are examples of the quality of the people we trained.

For a while I kept my staff position at Reese, but after a time it became evident that I could not perform satisfactory duties at both institutions. I left Reese, and began a ten-year full-time service at the University of Chicago.

At that time, the textbooks on neurology were not very good. My teaching in neurology was handicapped by the fact that, although the students attended courses in neuroanatomy, neurophysiology, and neuropathology, each area was taught separately and was not integrated with the others. When it came to clinical neurology, I had to teach the badly needed anatomy all over again.

At the faculty neurological club, I came into contact with

many illustrious figures who were working in the neurosciences at the University of Chicago: C.J. Herrick, G. Barthelmetz, Anton Carlson, Arno Luckhart, Karl S. Lashley, G.E. Coghill, C.M. Childs, R. Lillie, and R.W. Gerard. I was in awe of them, and I listened to them very carefully.

In the early twentieth century, this small group of naturalists working on animal experiments at the University of Chicago developed a series of process propositions on which many current concepts in psychiatry are based. Briefly, they stated that hypothetical whole living organisms function not simply as sums of their parts, but subserve new emergent functions; organisms mature by differentiation of primary undifferentiated structure-functions; living boundary structures are semipermeable and permit control of input and output; substructures of whole organisms exist in gradients under central control or regulation; Jackson's final common pathways carry many processes from divergent internal sources to achieve near-identical actions; and living organisms maintain homeostasis within a healthy range under conditions of moderate stress. These propositions were the precursors of what Ludwig von Bertalanffy (1968) was to describe much later as *general systems theory.*

I proposed that we transcend departmental lines in the teaching of the nervous system, that when a student was exposed to a particular anatomical system, for example, the physiologist could bring in experimental animals that were prepared to show disturbances of function of that system, and the clinicians could bring in a human with a disturbance of function from disease that was similar, thus accomplishing a *set* or synthesis at the beginning.

This, however, turned out to be impossible, because it required crossing departmental lines that were jealously guarded. Only in our neurological club could such interdisciplinary interchanges take place, so I decided to write a textbook. My book, now in its seventh edition, synthesized the neurosciences with clinical neurology as well as it could be done in the early days (1934). (Later, I had help from Bucy and Sahs, and the recent seventh edition of the book has been rewritten by Vick (1976).

The problem of synthesis attempted in the first volume was given up in the fourth edition, when superior textbooks of anatomy and physiology were finally being written, and there was no reason to include these sections. Thus, the book is not now like the first edition was intended to be.

In those days I worked with Bailey, saw all his patients, examined them, diagnosed them, and stood in the operating room while he opened their heads and removed their tumors. But the field was changing, and it was no longer fun or exciting to be a clinical neurologist—at least not as exciting as I had thought.

"Should I become a neurosurgeon?" I thought. No, I decided, my hands just could not do that. Now what about psychiatry? What should I do in this crucial phase of my life? I was making little money at the University of Chicago as an associate professor. I think I received $7,000 and some income from my parents' estate, which disappeared during the Great Depression. How could I support my family while changing specialties? Finally, while I struggled with my decision, Dean McLean surprised me by asking, "How would you like to go into psychiatry and establish a department here?" I answered, "I don't know if I *can.*" He said, "If you put in the energy and interest as you have in neurology, *you will.*" I only learned much later that this had been planned by Dr. McLean and various committees in correspondence between 1929 and 1932.

I was not happy about the opportunity. I remembered the boring lectures on psychiatry that I had attended in medical school; my roommate David Levy's statistical approaches; a sterile internship devoted only to diagnoses; Gordon Holmes's anger at neurotic patients at Queens Square, London; and Monakow's antipsychiatric quarrel with Eugene Bleuler in Zurich, but I accepted the opportunity. The career that followed is the essence of this book.

CHAPTER 2

Student and Analysand: A Career Begins

After much soul-searching and consultation with many colleagues, I decided to accept a Rockefeller Fellowship in Psychiatry, arranged by Dean McLean to begin at the end of the summer of 1932. Before leaving Chicago, I hurried to finish my neurology textbook. As I left, I cleaned out my bookshelves, put my gear in storage, and placed on my desk the manuscript—1,700 pages—that was to be the first edition. There were over 1,000 illustrations. I took a last look. I picked it up in my hands, threw it down on the desk, and said (thinking of my father, who had been so much the source of my struggles to achieve), "I hope you're satisfied!"

In 1932 there was no psychiatric department at the University of Chicago. Patients requiring psychiatrists were referred to one of several private practitioners downtown, a small group, in fact, since there were only about thirty-five psychiatrists in the state of Illinois, and most of them made a living practicing neurology.

Franz Alexander had been invited in 1931 to become a member of the University of Chicago faculty as a visiting professor, at the suggestion of a member of the social science faculty who had been analyzed by him in Berlin. He agreed to come only if he were made a visiting professor in the Department of Medicine. His stipulation was accepted, and he was required to give a course of lectures. At his first lecture before a body of distinguished internists, physiologists, and biochemists, he talked about a constipated female patient who was cured when her husband took Alexander's advice and brought his wife a bouquet of roses!

Pandemonium broke out. There was no opportunity for Alexander to say anything for the rest of the meeting. A memo from the dean—"There will be no further discussions until the end of all the seminar meetings"—deprived the Alexander lectures of most of their audience. So Alexander left Chicago for Boston, returning one year later to found the Chicago Institute for Psychoanalysis with the financial help of an enlightened Chicago businessman, Alfred Stern.

Psychiatry was, of course, only in its infancy, and there was much evidence that the medical profession was far from accepting it. I remember an incident that shattered the peace of the psychiatric community. When a medical student was hired as a "yard boy" by a professor on the University of Chicago faculty, he was asked why he needed such a job. He answered that the money was necessary to pay for his analytic fees. When this was reported to the medical school, a violent eruption ensued: The tradition was that physicians and medical students should be given free treatment by other doctors, and the fact that the many weekly analytic sessions often lasted for years was neither understood nor appreciated.

There were no psychiatric residencies of any stature in the United States at that time. The University of Pennsylvania graduate school had a regimented three-year course in psychiatry, but I felt it was preferable to pick and choose my "curriculum" for myself, so I began to read extensively. I wanted to read something about Freud, but none of his books were in the medical library. Finally I did find some—locked in the back room of the psychology library—and they had to be read right there. The librarian was careful about who read those books about sex, and they were returned to the locked case after each borrower had finished perusing them. I read this stuff, and the reason I got excited about it—not knowing the least thing about what the whole theory meant—was that I saw in some of the theoretical propositions of psychoanalysis a close analogy to Jacksonian neurology.

I saw that part structures, as they developed, were eventually organized and held down by supraordinate mechanisms, always maintaining, however, the capacity for revival of function if the organizer was disturbed, destroyed, or defective in any way. I saw the developmental stages in psychoanalysis as being similar.

Psychoanalytic regression and devolution in the Jacksonian sense were really the same process. It was then that I decided that I would immediately be psychoanalyzed, despite the admonitions of Herrick and Lashley.

I first contacted S. Ferenczi in Hungary, who unfortunately died during the course of our communications. Alexander then asked, "Why don't you go directly to Freud?" He wrote to Freud, but Freud said that he did not want to take me on because it would interfere with my academic career. It did not.

I began to write to Freud myself. The following are some excerpts from his correspondence, which I donated to the Freud Archives:

> Dear Dr. Grinker:
>
> You are right to assume that my greedy instincts will be strongly influenced by your future career in America. [I was truthfully pleading poverty.] But in addition there are material needs to be considered. I am still forced to make a living. I cannot do more than five hours of analysis daily; and I do not know how much longer I shall work at it. I can make no other arrangements." [That was in May.]
>
> [In June] I am glad to hear that it has been made easier for you to be in analysis with me since I myself care about it. The first of September would be a good time to start. As concerns the fee, you are rather too discrete about it, which is unjustified among analysts. You mention no figure. I do not recall whether I made you a positive proposal. I think I only illustrated the shortcomings of your calculations. Also the circumstances have changed since. The dollar has lost much of its value and perhaps will drop further within the next few months.

The financial question was resolved when the Rockefeller Foundation and the University of Chicago agreed to pay twenty-five dollars in American money per hour for my analysis. I also managed to have some money left over to pay for my living expenses. I might say at this point that the belief that a financial sacrifice is necessary for a successful analysis was denied by Freud himself. He offered Paul Schilder a free analysis if he would stay in Vienna and not go to America. He also offered Hartmann a free analysis, and I know that Hartmann accepted it.

A flood of Freud anecdotes and reminiscences come to mind. After my first session with him, his daughter Anna called me to say he was sick. As a matter of fact, he had broncho-pneumonia. I thought—in the magical way that analysands think—that perhaps it was I who had made him sick. I was full of anxiety, waiting for his return, which occurred in about three weeks. Finally, we resumed the analysis.

In his office, there was a couch with a linen doily at the head end and a comfortable armchair behind. Next to his chair was a reflector light, but there was no plug in the wall, so that the cord was stretched to the source of electricity on the opposite side of the room.

Freud was very much interested in geography, and any time the name of a town or a city was mentioned, he would get up and go to the second room, where he kept various figures made of ivory and little statuettes on his working desk. One day, when I had mentioned a certain town, he got up to consult an atlas. But in doing so he tripped and fell over the electric cord, hitting his nose and bloodying it. And there I was, lying on the couch with Professor Freud lying on the floor with a bloody nose. It took me a while to recover from that!

It is most difficult in any transference to express hostility to a genius. I couldn't tell Freud certain things I thought about him; I had to use certain indirections. For instance, I used to study in a beer hall with Jake Finesinger. We would go over the original German of Freud's entire writings as if we were studying the Talmud. Jake was not being analyzed, and as he read the stuff that he could not understand, he used to call Freud all kinds of names. In my analysis I found I could quote Finesinger's negative remarks: I did not say those things; Jake did. Eventually, Margaret Gerard joined us, but not for long, because she and Finesinger did not get along.

I could also scold the dog, which was definitely involved in my analysis and in that way indirectly express my hostility to Freud. When I rang the bell of the door which opened onto the waiting room that both the Professor and Anna utilized, there would be a horrendous barking from the other side. Paula, the maid, would open the door and a great big wolfhound would attack me with its snout at the same level as my genitalia. So, I entered Freud's office with a high level of castration anxiety.

At one of the child psychiatric seminars that Anna held for the Americans, somehow or other that damn dog lay down next to my chair and started to bark. Anna said, "Dr. Grinker, he's perfectly safe. Of course, when he was younger, he used to eviscerate sheep, and I couldn't take him out. But now he's perfectly safe; just pull his tail and he'll stop barking." Not me!

In Freud's own office there was also another dog, a Chinese chow named Jofi. Jofi would sit alongside the couch, and after a while got up and scratch at the door to be let out. The Professor would get up, let the dog out, and come back and say, "Jofi doesn't approve of what you're saying." Then, after a while, the dog would scratch at the other side of the door, and the Professor would get up, open the door, and say, "Jofi wants to give you another chance."

In this country, no candidate would continue for long under these conditions! Once when I was emoting with a great deal of vigor, the dog jumped on top of me, and Freud said, "You see, Jofi is so excited that you've been able to discover the source of your anxiety." But I wasn't paying the dog!

I sometimes mentioned to Freud my difficulty in understanding transference. One night my wife and I were invited to the house of young Dr. Sippy from Chicago who was being analyzed in Vienna. His wife, who I found out later was being analyzed by Anna Freud, was also at the party. We had quite a social evening, and, at an appropriate occasion, I told a joke that Freud had told me. At the next session, Freud said to me, "I thought we decided that this analysis was confidential." I had thought the confidential part was on his side, not on mine. To my surprise, I burst into tears at his criticism. And he said, "Well, now you know what transference is."

Many analysands worry as to whether their analysts are going to sleep during their sessions, but they never have the courage to look. I looked, however, and as far as I know, Freud never did go to sleep during my analysis. When he was ready to make an interpretation that he thought was quite fitting and related to uncovering some important material, he would become excited and would pound the edge of the couch. As he talked, the prosthesis in his mouth would make him salivate, and the saliva would cover my face. Every time my face was covered with saliva, I knew that I was making progress in my analysis.

Sometimes I became quite irritated. I learned one day that an assistant of Freud's at the publishing company had died of Landry's ascending paralysis, a neurological disease not well known in Vienna. I knew what the disease was, but I did not know what caused it. Freud wanted to know all about it. I tried to get off the subject, but I had to spend the whole hour talking about Landry's paralysis rather than about myself, who should have been the center of attention.

Every time Dr. O'Brien, the European chief for the Rockefeller Foundation, came to Vienna, he would take my wife and me out to dinner and to a movie. On one visit, he wanted an interview with Freud. I said I would try to arrange it, but Freud refused to see him. I said, "Well, he can have one of my hours. After all, the Rockefeller Foundation is paying for this, so why shouldn't he have an interview?" "Absolutely not," he replied. "When I needed help for my publishing house and applied to the Rockefeller Foundation, I was turned down, and I will not see him."

This incident brings up an attribute of Freud's that is generally recognized—he never forgot and rarely forgave. This characteristic was reflected in his attitude toward Americans as a group. There were three important causes for his hostility. One was the fact that Jung had written to him that if he soft-pedaled the sexual aspects of psychoanalytic theory, the Americans would accept psychoanalysis more quickly. Freud responded in the negative: If psychoanalysis was diluted too much, it would cease to be psychoanalysis. The second reason for his dislike of Americans was President Wilson's failure to put over the fourteen points he had promised the Europeans because of the Senate's obstructionism toward the League of Nations. The third was a reaction to what he saw was a lack of concern for *him*. When he was at Putnam's camp in the Adirondacks, he developed intestinal cramps with diarrhea and felt very sick. When people there would ask him how he felt, he replied that he did not feel well at all. "That's too bad," they said, and walked on. Freud never forgave them for their lack of interest.

In 1940, on Freud's birthday, I gave a paper that was later published in the *Orthogenic Journal,* discussing Freud's dislike of Americans and the reasons for it. I also indicated that even geniuses can make mistakes, that we must not ask perfection of Freud any more than of any human being. There was no response to this publication until thirty-three years later, when it was included in *Freud As We Knew Him* (Ruitenbeek, 1973). After that, I received several letters from readers through the *Journal of the American Psychiatric Association* accusing me of libel.

One of Freud's favorite techniques was the frequent use of metaphors. He always had some story to tell that exemplified an interpretation. He had anecdotes about everything. His stories made things extraordinarily clear. Freud knew of my fondness for a woman in Vienna who was extremely intelligent. He had also obtained a good deal of information about my wife from his daughter. It was a sneaky bit of dealing, but he did it. He accepted what was generally known by most people, that my wife was an extraordinarily beautiful and charming woman. But the other woman was a very intelligent professional, and I liked to talk to her as I did to intelligent men.

Freud told me a story about a man who loved to hear a particular wind instrument. One day, when an artist on this particular instrument came to town, he took his son to hear the man play. He turned to his son and said, "Doesn't this sound just like a violin?" And the son answered, "Why don't we go listen to a violin, then?"

After about three months of our stay in Vienna, my wife said, "I don't believe you're telling him everything." I said, "Well, why don't you? Why don't you write to him?" I mentioned this to Freud and he said, "Yes, let her write to me, providing she doesn't expect me to answer the letter." So my wife sat down and wrote three pages of accusations and these of course entered into my analysis.

About two or three months later, for some reason or other which I did not suspect at the time, names of distant people kept creeping into my wife's conversation. Apparently my responses were no different, so my wife decided to write another letter to

Freud. "See here, Professor Freud, it's been three months since I've written to you, about my husband's attitude, and I see no change. Why don't you do something?" That was probably the first time he had ever received such a correspondence. Unfortunately, we had no carbon copies of these letters. I later asked Anna Freud if she could send me copies. Here is her answer:

> Dear Dr. Grinker,
>
> Thank you for your letter of March 9th.
>
> I am very sorry, but the letters of your wife to my father are not with me. When we left Vienna, only a certain selection of letters came with us and many others had to stay behind. I feel very sorry that I cannot fulfill your request.
>
> Yours sincerely,
> Anna Freud

My wife wanted to be aware of what I was going to be doing in the future, and so she decided she should begin to see an analyst. I did not have very much money, so I went to Helene Deutsch and asked if she could recommend an analyst for her that would not be too expensive. She did, and it turned out to be Siegfried Bernfeld, one of the most erudite and one of the most knowledgeable, most effective people in the field. After a trial period, he said to her, "I think you need an analysis."

We were fortunate in that we were accepted into the social group of the Vienna analysts. Every Saturday night we were at one of the houses of the Bibrings', or the Deutschs' or the Waelders' or the Krises' or even the Hartmanns', occasionally. We had supper and we talked. I suspected that they wanted to increase their knowledge of English, but, at any rate, it was a pleasant social existence. I loved Helene Deutsch. In fact, she became a way in which I expressed my hostilities to Freud, because I told him repeatedly that I had made a mistake and should have gone to Helene Deutsch. She would not have said such things as he was saying to me.

I brought Freud a story about cigars. A story was circulating around Vienna that when he could not smoke cigars anymore because of his cancer, he would light a cigar and waft the smoke up his nostrils in order to enjoy the smell. This he denied flatly. And then I added, "But I can't find a good cigar in all of Vienna."

He got up from his chair, went to his desk, opened a box, brought a cigar, and gave it to me. I wrapped that cigar in tissue paper. I never smoked it. I kept it until it crumbled into pieces.

The German our children quickly picked up included the Viennese dialect, and they feigned their astonishment when we pronounced words correctly. My son correctly assumed that the purpose of my sessions with Freud was to tell him what a bad boy I had been. The children did well in public school, but were frightened of the principal with his bass voice and their governess who demanded perfection in their homework. At age five, my son thought that his future source of livelihood would be in cashing American Express® travelers' checks, but he later studied at the University of Chicago and Harvard Medical School, and then had a psychiatric residency at Reese. During that time I refrained from teaching there for several years. He unfortunately forgot all the German he had learned, but he became a psychiatrist and analyst—excellent in both fields.

I studied analysis seriously. I also went to the psychiatric clinic headed by Poetzl and Hans Hoff, for whom I had no regard. Freud permitted me to attend conferences and seminars and meetings of the analytic society, though ordinarily this was not permitted. I used to bring him stories concerning the emotionality, in fact, rages, of people who were supposed to be thoroughly analyzed, but as Freud said, "They are still human." When I commented to Freud that one of his long-term patients shrieked and cried as she left his office before my turn he said, "You should have seen her before." To my surprise and gratification, Freud's last words to me were: "Your psychoanalysis was one of my few last remaining pleasures."

After leaving Vienna in 1935 I traveled through Germany to visit the great universities, which seemed to be destined for destruction in the impending holocaust. I found a secret interest in psychoanalysis there, but the young psychiatrists had to hide all books written by Freud. In 1968, on a trip through West Germany for the Foundations Fund for Research in Psychiatry (FFRP), I again found the old-style neuropsychiatry, though there were some young female clinical psychologists studying Kleinian psychoanalysis.

As I have already suggested, my first years back at the University of Chicago were most unfulfilling because the university had not yet entered the world of modern psychiatry. I wrote to Freud about my frustrations, because he had predicted that analysis would ruin my academic year. But, in fact, his misgivings were not quite accurate. It was not analysis that was the problem, but the university medical school itself. When he heard about my leaving the university, he expressed his surprise:

> Dear Dr. Grinker:
>
> I was somewhat surprised by the news. I had assumed that you had a secure position at the University. Now that you've turned away from the strictly academic career, I may hope that analysis has made a valuable catch, which I prefer it this way. I suspect that you will be as satisfied in the end. With many kind regards to you and your wife.

It was impossible to remain at the University of Chicago Medical School with its antagonism to psychiatry and harrassing obstacles. When a delegation from Michael Reese Hospital came in 1937 to invite me back, I accepted with alacrity, although the separation was not easy. In 1939, I was able to set up a small psychiatric inpatient unit at Reese, but I felt compelled to enlist in the Air Force for service overseas. In 1942, during World War II, I joined my ex-resident, John Spiegel. Overseas and later, in Florida, we wrote our treatise on war neuroses, entitled *Men Under Stress.*

CHAPTER 3

The Return to Civilian Life: A New Psychiatric Institute Is Founded

MY EXPERIENCE as a military psychiatrist during World War II was to have a lasting effect on my interests and on the course of my professional career. The return to civilian life was not an easy transition. My colleagues and I suffered some of the same "culture shocks" as many of the soldiers, sailors, and airmen who had experienced combat. It was especially difficult for the medical officers to adapt themselves to postwar life—many were seriously depressed and resented the financial and professional advantages that had come to those colleagues who had been privileged to spend the war years at home.

On November 11, 1946, a group of military psychiatrists, furious at the older members of the American Psychiatric Association who had abandoned them to the imbecilities of the military medical hierarchy, established a progressive new society called The Group for the Advancement of Psychiatry (GAP) (Deutsch, 1959). It was a small group composed of several committees.

In 1966, on the twentieth anniversary of GAP, I wrote an editorial essay sketching its early history:

> In 1946 a group of military psychiatrists recently returnd to civilian life, decided to form an organization designed to put new life into the American Psychiatric Association, which had let its colleagues fight their professional battles with the military unaided and had slothfully avoided any position of real leadership. The new organization was not to be rebellious or a substitute for the old, but a constructive influence stimulating from within. By means of its committee organization, two yearly meetings, and continuous work at home, members of this Group for the Advancement of Psychiatry (GAP) studied many topical issues and published significant reports distrib-

uted and appreciated the world over. American psychiatry was stimulated and the American Psychiatric Association was modernized, but GAP could not disband because it continues to serve important purposes that organized psychiatry cannot. It is destined to remain for many years to come, and to resolve many significant issues through scholarly deliberations.

An example of this function could be observed at the plenary session on November 11, 1966, when two speakers discussed the role of psychiatry in the modern Great Society. Dr. Bertram Brown, late deputy director of The National Institute for Mental Health, commanded us to direct our attention to the many problems of our rapidly changing world. His speech, with its repetitive "musts" called our attention to the psychiatric needs and implications of juvenile delinquency, narcotic addiction, mental deficiency, forensic psychiatry, urban renewal, community psychiatry, and suicide prevention, etc. We were informed that we "must" participate and advise in the development of the new "guidelines" that were in the making or were being planned.

The next speaker, Dr. Walter Barton, spoke quietly and soberly with the voice of knowledge and experience and with a full understanding of current needs. Representing GAP, his spirit had not dulled by the years into misunderstanding the tone of contemporary fervor. He emphasized the primary role of the physician-psychiatrist in treating the sick, disturbed, or deviant by individual, family, or group methods, whether the person is a child, an adolescent, an adult, or senile. He emphasized that contemporary psychiatrists need to understand environmental or sociocultural processes, just as the general physician has done from antiquity. We are not magicians, he reminded us, or social engineers, but physicians and scientists, nor can we wishfully divide by simple fission (cloning) into multiples of ourselves to create the necessary manpower, nor will we be content to adopt a role as consultants and supervisors to subprofessionals or "expediters."

It is clear that the issues to which Dr. Barton addressed himself in 1966 are for the most part the same ones with which we are grappling today. We cannot be all things to all societies, cultures, or "catchment areas." But is it not important to know where we are going and the pathways we should take? Are there not pilot programs to investigate before we sacrifice our heritages for an exhilarating ride on a bandwagon? Is it not possible to develop feedback systems of evaluation within any new enterprise and not assume that thought and plan are synonymous with successful action? Should we not finally come to grips with the question of what we actually accomplish with whatever technique we use for the treatment of any age-group or kind of disturbance? Are we as doctors of the mind getting worthwhile results? If we do not achieve "tertiary prevention," and if "secondary prevention" is a myth, then maybe we had better just try to prevent, even if nobody knows how. The try may be valuable.

My questions as yet have no answers, but perhaps GAP may slowly, through dignified scholarly discussions and much careful thinking, produce some answers or perhaps even better questions. It may even be possible to develop harmony from apparent discordance! I am gratified that GAP is still alive and well, and functioning at a high level of sophistication.

One of the most significant events in the immediate postwar period was the establishment in 1946 of the National Institute for Mental Health (NIMH). Mr. and Mrs. Albert D. Lasker of New York were largely instrumental in its founding. They were people who were always more interested in broad social issues than in individual projects. Sometimes, in fact, their efforts were highly misguided. They believed, for example, that the new drugs or lobotomies advertised in the 1950s (the Russians were the first to abandon the latter) were the only, and the final, solution for the cure of mental illness. For a long time, those who did not subscribe to this laymen's notion of cure were ignored when NIMH funds were distributed.

I became a member of the Research Study Group of the National Institute for Mental Health, a committee that in the course of the years divided into many study sections. Eventually, I was chairman of the program-project section, and later of the psychopharmological section. In the early years, we had little money, and few grant requests included the names of investigators. As a result, the first meetings of this illustrious group, chaired by the competent John Romano, were devoted to making rules that would protect the professionals from interference from the bureaucrats. We were successful for several years, but gradually the executive secretaries of each section and the lay members of the supraordinate council took over. This is really a pity!

My main activity during these years was to plan and raise money for the new Psychiatric and Psychosomatic Institute at Michael Reese. Although Mr. Lasker was a major donor, he did not want the building to bear his name, for fear of discouraging other donors in the future. I was certain that I did not want a fifty-bed hospital devoid of teaching and research space, as the current medical director had projected. One of our first tasks was to choose an architect. After many interviews we chose Loebl (whom I had known as a youngster), Schlossman, and later Bennett, who had never before built a hospital. Reginald Isaacs was hired as consultant. He was a progressive young man who was an architectural graduate of Harvard. He insisted on large, airy rooms and wide corridors with windows at both ends.

Though the building turned out to be both beautiful and efficient, it was not as well maintained as it should have been, and twenty-five years of use have brought us to the point where today rehabilitation of our facilities is absolutely necessary. It is difficult in times of economic stringency to realize that deterioration must be constantly fought and corrected. To do less is shortsighted, to say the least. Current rehabilitation is likely to cost as much as $5 million.

In planning the new building, we took plenty of time. Our goals expanded and our costs mounted, though we were constantly reassured by Mr. Schwarz, the chairman of the board of trustees, that we must plan the best possible building, regardless of cost. The final cost was $1.6 million. The money was raised, and the Institute was built.

But what a struggle! I was attacked by those who felt I was depriving the Israelis of needed money to fight the Arabs. Others asked why money should be spent on psychiatry when medical and surgical beds were needed. There were other priorities competing for the hospital's money and attention: The first long tunnel from Main Reese to the new building—part of a system built to serve all the new buildings on the campus—was constructed at a cost of $400,000. The ghetto neighborhood around the hospital had to be torn down and its occupants relocated if the hospital was to survive in its present location and not be forced to move to a high-rise complex.

During our first six months, we operated at a deficit because the doctors were slow in using the institute as a resource for their patients. The board of trustees of the Jewish Federation called me on the carpet and suggested that we give up. I fought back angrily and was given another six months. The going was rough. Many of our staff members were admitting patients without professional charge, even though hospital costs were then only twenty-five dollars per day. Some of the Reese staff stood at the tunnel excavation, calling it "Grinker's Gulch." Others stood in front of our entrance waiting to take over our rooms. But, within a year, we were on our feet—and our solvency and our success have continued.

In 1951, we moved to our new institute with five nurses from our previous quarters in First Meyer House, each to become a head nurse of a division. A chief nurse had been employed to set up a loose-leaf operational manual, which was constantly modified and has been kept in use throughout the years. In the meantime, the interest of the Lasker family waned, and after a while they did not even contribute to the annual Lasker Memorial Lecture, which we continued to support on our own until 1970, when we funded an endowment for the Grinker Lectureship in perpetuity.

I must admit that I opened the institute with some trepidation. There was a constant fear that we would not make it. I had a terrible feeling that now no alibi was possible. People who have little money and poor quarters, few instruments, and few assistants can always provide excuses about what they *could have done,* but when I walked into the new institute in June 1951 I realized that we had no choice but to succeed.

To commemorate the opening of our new institute, we organized a day of scientific discussions, which I later edited under the title *Mid-Century Psychiatry* (1953a). Among the contributors were Percival Bailey, Ralph Gerard, George Engel, Therese Benedek, David Shakow, Howard Liddell, David Levy, M. Ralph Kaufman, Thomas French, Charles Johnson, Franz Alexander, and John Spiegel. The preface to the book expressed the hopes and the purposes of the new institute.

On June 1, 1951, the Institute for Psychosomatic and Psychiatric Research and Training (P & PI) of Michael Reese Hospital was dedicated by a gathering of scientists who spoke on varying aspects of midcentury psychiatry. Their contributions are recorded as contemporary statements and promises of several disciplines that have contributed greatly to the science of behavior. This symposium, far from indicating that the twentieth midcentury was close to producing the awaited synthesis of many disciplines into a behavioral science, emphasized the absence of a basic or unitary concept of human nature, the polyglot nature of interdisciplinary communications, and the failure of diverse and multileveled operational procedures to permit sound correlations. Today, however, there are many signs indicating that these goals are understood with greater clarity and that many are engaged in positive efforts to attain them despite huge obstacles.

Our condition at P & PI was indeed precarious, and the early struggle for existence required my constant attention. I went to the hospital on Saturdays and Sundays as well as weekdays, supervising everyone, in order to mold an efficient operation. This prevented me from accepting an offer to participate in the Center for study of the Behavioral Sciences in Palo Alto, California.

The skeleton staff of psychiatrists and partly trained nurses with which we began in 1951 in the new building created an extremely difficult task for me. But it was exciting to meet the challenge and to realize that the goal was worth the effort to overcome all of the obstacles. The end results clearly depended on our skill in selecting staff, our dedication to their education, and our continued stimulation of their morale. At times, the job seemed impossible; at other times, there were great satisfactions.

The five separate nursing units we established included one for disturbed patients, another for children, and a third for psychosomatic cases. The children's unit was badly managed, due partly to our fantasy that a hospital nursing unit could substitute for a residential treatment center for children. After five years (in 1956) we had to close the unit, an act that aroused great repercussions among the agencies from which our referrals had come.

The psychosomatic unit was a failure because it was naïve and premature to expect that in the 1950s and 1960s patients suffering from illnesses they considered "medical" would enter a psychiatric hospital.

Social workers, young psychiatrists, and nurses required close supervision, even after their formal training was completed. Several posts required especially careful control: the positions of clinical director, assistant director of the institute, chief of the outpatient service, chief nurse, chief of psychiatric social workers, director of psychology, and chief of liaison psychiatry. The personnel holding these positions tended to change somewhat rapidly, either because they were not competent enough, or because those who were competent wanted a higher position with greater perstige and a higher salary. No job was static—change was prevalent. Eventually we settled down, especially when we developed separate peer groups for adolescents, young adults, middle adults, and elderly (geriatric) patients. The staff consisted of only a few salaried, full-time psychiatrists; most were unpaid voluntary physicians in private practice. Recently, consultants to the search committee organized to find a replacement for me commented on how impressed they were with the large number of voluntary staff members who satisfactorily filled full-time staff positions. They had obviously remained because of gratitude for their education and a loyalty to the educational institution that had trained them; they resisted leaving for any other institution.

My credo for the new institute sets forth the principles that have guided it over the past two and one-half decades. It was originally presented at a banquet held on the evening of our dedication. Later, it was enlarged in scroll form and placed over the front desk in the Institute lobby. It continues to set forth our goals as an institution dedicated to the service of humankind:

> May our assumptions be undistorted and faithful to the proven labors of our scientific predecessors.
>
> May the questions we ask of nature be reasonable and appropriate to the principles of unitary man.
>
> May our powers of observation be sharp and our technique of measurement accurate.

May we have the breadth of knowledge to include in our study of behavior all possible help from the concepts, operational methods, and knowledge of many disciplines of science.

May our emphasis on understanding human behavior not lead us to neglect any level of biological activity properly identified, nor confuse several levels in false correlations.

May we strive for originality, freedom of imagination, and the courage to leave the highway for new and unbroken paths toward our goals.

May we never become structuralized in our concepts, ritualized in our procedures, or formalized in our therapies.

May we ever strive to transmit clearly without pride our knowledge, and with humility the fields of our ignorance to the eager, curious students of all fields.

May we strive to apply our learning to the preservation of health and the treatment of illness.

May the promise and hope of this Institute be transmitted without decrement to many generations of young, fresh, and enthusiastic workers to whom we shall give unrestricted opportunities for help and progress.

CHAPTER 4

Psychiatry in the 1950s and 1960s: Changes in Treatment, Education, and Research

IT HAS OFTEN seemed that psychiatry is becoming as broad as life itself. So many applications and extensions of the field have come and gone that it has been difficult for students to maintain their composure amidst the current controversies or for patients to choose their physicians intelligently. The old organic approaches that depended on drugs such as bromides and phenobarbital had given way before the great promises of psychoanalysis or of the shorter kinds of psychoanalytic psychotherapy.

The long-time adherence to individual therapy has been diluted by emphasis on groups, family, psychopharmacology, short-term psychotherapy, community psychiatry, behavioral therapy, psychotherapy, and encounter groups of all degrees of bizarreness. Semireligions and Oriental cults have developed therapeutic garbs. Conflict and argument have developed between the so-called medical and humanistic models of psychiatry. Therapeutic *peer groups* (*see* Chap. 12), consisting of children, adolescents, young adults, middle-aged adults, and geriatric patients; are separated in the hospitals and treated with different techniques. Yet, systems of evaluation and sound data concerning effectiveness are still lacking. The success of any particular style of therapy is difficult to measure, although Strupp (1973) has valiantly tried to do so over the years. The variables are too difficult to control. This is discussed later in more detail.

At Michael Reese, our training program (a better term would be *education*) began after the war, in 1946, with a group of ten residents, in contrast to our earlier, prewar organization of two resident pairs. Eventually, we admitted seven, not very well generally educated (now half of them are female) residents per year to be trained as general psychiatrists in an eclectic institute. As psychiatry became extended, we had to include more and more subject matter, making it necessary to provide an increasing degree of specialization. The need soon arose for more space. To some degree, our increased requirements were met by the new Wexler Pavilion for clinic outpatients, a facility that was especially helpful when our laboratories had to be given up.

Social workers, who after the war were used as "junior psychotherapists," required considerable time for effective staff development. From 1925 to 1949, our social service students came from Smith College—later, they were drawn from the University of Chicago School of Social Service Administration.

The evolution of the social worker from the "friendly visitor" to the professional specialist was slow and tortuous (Grinker, MacGregor, Selan, Klein, and Kohrman, 1961). At each phase of the specialty's growth, its practitioners were doubtful and insecure, constantly searching for certainty. Conflicts between academic teachers of social work theory and practical chiefs of psychiatric services, who needed as much therapeutic time for their overwhelming case loads as possible, resulted in a victory for the chiefs of service. Social workers moved gradually from casework to depth psychology and psychotherapy. But the "pied pipers" of psychodynamics and psychotherapy led them into dangerously deep waters and more confusion and ambiguity.

Today, the pendulum is slowly swinging back toward a more sophisticated view of the "social" aspects of the social worker's functions. The social worker has a revived interest in the family and an interest in family therapy. He or she speaks bravely of the "social matrix of psychiatry" from which clients develop, but recognizes that they ultimately are likely to remain, or return, to function as psychiatric practitioners. Staff development is facilitated not only through seminars conducted by psychiatrists, but also through exposure to the knowledge and theory of modern social science. More than ever, social workers are becoming aware of a specific professional identity.

Danger still exists; in fact, it currently is becoming intense, that social work may become arrested at the level of theory and concepts, to the neglect of the practical. The brief history of psychiatric social work reveals that the socialwork practice has tended to take supremacy over theoretical academic teaching expounded in many schools. Before predictions can be made about what new directions will be taken in the future, it is important to more clearly assess the role of social work today. It is hoped that these questions can be answered, in order to clarify the present status of the profession and, as a result, to sharpen its vision for the future. Of one thing we are sure: The social worker will not become a social engineer!

In addition to our efforts to integrate social workers into our treatment team at P & PI, we conducted a psychosomatic clinic staffed by internists under supervision, but we soon discovered that the transference problems were too sticky. We then began a system of liaison psychiatry, with many in– and outpatient services. When the demand for this service became too great, we had to rely on the responding departments to carry part-time psychiatrists on their own departmental budgets.

The most troublesome group to incorporate into our program were the clinical psychologists. We were fortunate, finally, in being able to obtain Martin Harrow from Yale, who organized an excellent predoctoral training program and became an integral part of our schizophrenic research team, contributing many good research papers that were published in significant journals. Though for years I had resisted the idea of permitting therapeutic roles for clinical psychologists, finally I had to give in. At the present time, psychologists as well as social workers treat patients with various methods of psychotherapy.

Psychologists were also accepted for two-year postdoctoral fellowships, until their demand for equality with the psychiatric residents became excessive, and they began to expect the right to have private offices, treat inpatients, and write prescriptions. We then took only psychology interns who were preparing to study for advanced degrees. We found this group less arrogant and more eager to learn.

Our ancillary professional personnel were both helpful and troublesome. Nevertheless, we worked hard to integrate them into the program as successfully as possible and to keep them fully apprised of our goals and purposes.

As we began to work toward medical affiliation with the University of Chicago, we realized that it would be necessary to assume the added burden of teaching the principles of psychiatry to half the class. In 1969, we began this chore, and our efforts were so successful that university students soon fought for assignment to our services.

Research began at P & PI, as it had ended in the military service, in a continuing interest in stress stimuli, in the responses of free anxiety, and in serious physiological disturbances—the latter an interest that grew out of my concern about the importance of synthesizing. By 1977, members of the institute had published 560 papers. From 1946 to 1960, my own interest was in larger programs, such as stress effects, response specificity, coping, and depression. From 1960 to 1970, I studied normality, diagnostic classification, the borderline syndrome, and general systems or unified theory. In the 1970s, with Philip Holzman, a large and lengthy study of schizophrenia was begun, and Harrow, Koh, Walsh, Schwartz, and Apter later joined the research team in this activity, which will far outlast me.

In 1951, with support from the Carnegie Corporation through the cooperation of John Gardner, we established a multidisciplinary group that met twice a year for five years to discuss a unified theory of human behavior. Our findings were published (1947, 1956; paperback edition, 1967).

Our first peer group of adolescents began in 1957. In 1956, we deemphasized shock treatment and began to use the modern antipsychotic drugs. The details of change cannot be completely described, but some idea of the growing impact of pharmacology in treating mental illness may be obtained from the introductions I have written through the years to our annual reports.

From 1946 until the 1960s, psychiatry enjoyed its "golden years," with a good deal of financial support, as I have already mentioned, from the National Institute for Mental Health. Gradually, however, support weakened, and the private sector has not yet taken up the slack. Our institute received help from the government, at the state and federal levels, as well as from a women's organization known as the Chicago Mental Health Foundation, and from other "friends" of psychiatry who have contributed to our research over the years. Administration has become increasingly difficult, as government controls, regulations, and reports impinge endlessly on our resources and time. Federal bureacracies must be matched at the local level, causing administrative functions to proliferate and faceless committees to assume control of a multitude of operations. Thus, proud as I was that P & PI produced so many chairmen of psychiatric departments throughout the country, I eventually was doomed to disappointment, as such highly effective people as George Ham, David Hamburg, Melvin Sabshin, and others turned from research to administration.

There has been a further onslaught, as forensic problems and malpractice suits have required increasingly more specialized legal defenses. National medical organizations and associations have been forced to turn their attention from scientific advancement and discovery and the enhancement of medical care to defensive legal maneuvers, and, what is more, third-party payments have crippled our financial structure. We are furthermore being attacked from within and without, by critics such as Szasz and Torrey.

My own efforts to establish a consortium of Chicago psychiatric centers were blocked by the selfishness and parochialism of each of the participating schools, and my early enthusiasm and optimism inevitably changed to a pessimistic feeling of frustration and disappointment. Our local, regional, and national activities have become dominated by psychopolitics (Cavanaugh, 1978).

In the early 1960s, we realized that we could no longer continue to use the general clinic building for our outpatient services. We needed more space, a different layout, and longer hours, but, even more basically, we needed an administration that understood psychiatric problems. Against considerable opposition from the hospital medical board, I obtained seed money from Mrs. Simon Wexler, the widow of a good friend, for the building of a new facility in her husband's memory. With that start, I was able to obtain funds from the private sector and from the government for a round building attached to P & PI that would provide thirty-five offices and a ground-floor laboratory.

The award-winning building designed by the architects Gordon and Levin is the most beautiful building on our campus. It was dedicated in 1962 and has served P & PI well since then.

The first legal assault on the confidentiality of psychiatric records—of which I was aware—occurred in 1952, although, of course, the issue has attracted a good deal of attention since then. When the husband of one of my patients demanded to see her hospital record to facilitate a divorce action against her, I of course refused and thereby exposed myself to contempt of court. The judge finally ruled in my favor. The battle was then carried on by precedent until we were strong enough to carry the issue through the legislature (Binder v. Russell, Civil Document 52C 2535, Circuit Court of Cook County, June 24, 1952).

During the middle 1960s, it became apparent that biological research in psychiatry no longer held top priority. (The pendulum has now swung the other way.) Work in the study sections began to focus on issues relating to the human situation. Grants to competent behavioral scientists, psychophysiologists, and neurochemists were not renewed, but fortunately, these able researchers found other good positions. I had to convert the laboratories to clinical space suitable for teaching and for our extended schizophrenia research program.

In 1951, I was appointed to the editorial board of the *Archives of Neurology and Psychiatry,* with Dr. Tracy Putnam, a neurosurgeon, as a chief editor. It was in fact a neurological journal and had little to do with modern psychiatry. But, to my surprise, in 1956, the American Medical Association decided to split the *Archives of Neurology* from an *Archives Psychiatry,* and I was asked to be the new journal's chief editor. Although the editorship was designed to be held for only ten years, the AMA changed the name of the journal twice; thus, my position was actually extended for thirteen years. With the help of a supportive board of editors, I was able to develop the *Archives of General Psychiatry* into a journal that became known and respected the world over and has achieved the highest circulation of any psychiatric periodical.

The aims and purposes of the *Archives of General Psychiatry* were set forth in its first editorial, and I believe it would be worthwhile to quote it here:

AMA ARCHIVES OF GENERAL PSYCHIATRY

An important reason for the establishment of a new Archives devoted entirely to psychiatry is the realistic recognition that neuropsychiatry has become separated into neurology and psychiatry as distinct clinical specialties. Each group of specialists has been penalized by receiving an *Archives of Neurology and Psychiatry* of which only half interests it. Although it is true that the structure, function, and pathology of the central nervous system are significant aspects of the basic sciences necessary for the training and development of the broadly educated psychiatrist, the details of existing clinical neurological knowledge are of little interest or practical use, and are not remembered. It is, instead, the extrapolated broad principles that are of importance for the congruence of physiological and psychological functions. Certainly, the psychiatrist should read and understand current research leading to breakthroughs of existing barriers to proper understanding and treatment of the major psychoses, such as the newer psychopharmacology, as well as the selected basic advances in neurophysiology significant for the understanding of psychodynamics and psychopathology. These works we shall continue to publish.

We shall publish contributions from all disciplines, whether morphological, physiological, biochemical, endocrinological, psychosomatic, psychological, psychiatric, child-psychiatric, psychoanalytical, sociological, or anthropological, that are related to the study of the behavior of Man in health and illness. We shall attempt to implement the concept that Man's behavior cannot in our day be viewed profitably from a narrow frame of reference. Instead it requires a broad vision of a totally integrated field composed of many part functions and transactions, which constitute the focus of a wide variety of scientific disciplines. Eventually a *unified science of behavior* may emerge.

From the time of its inception, the editors of the *Archives of General Psychiatry* recognized that psychiatrists rarely carry on clinical research in isolation, but cooperate with psychologists, social workers, and other scientists. A vast number of nonmedical disciplines not only learn about personality and its disorders from psychiatrists, but in turn contribute greatly to advances in psychiatric knowledge. The psychiatric field is constantly increasing in breadth and depth, and it needs a forum for the many life disciplines that are concerned with its progress.

In the *Archives of General Psychiatry,* we published contributions from all disciplines related to the study of the behavior of man in health and illness—morphological, physiological, biochemical, endocrinological, psychosomatic, psychological, psychiatric, child psychiatric, psychoanalytical, sociological, or anthropological. We attempted to implement the concept that currently, man's behavior cannot be viewed profitably from a narrow frame of reference, but requires a broad vision of a totally integrated field composed of many part functions and transactions, each of which constitutes the focus of a wide variety of scientific disciplines. It is to be hoped that eventually a unified science, or system theory, of behavior may emerge.

That more scientific papers are written by doctors of philosophy than by medical doctors is a disturbing fact to those of us who would foster a scientific psychiatry. Papers submitted by psychiatrists tend to be long discursive essays presenting little or no data; though there are, of course, many exceptions, too few essays on topical subjects are appropriate and relevant summaries.

Although it was not the purpose of the *Archives of General Psychiatry* to dismiss psychodynamic principles or to reject psychotherapy based on these principles, we did, however, desire to extend and expand the psychiatric field, without sacrificing the dynamic point of view or alienating or losing its teachers. But such a policy created almost insurmountable resistances and brought us into a struggle for greater eclecticism.

A number of organic theories were briefly explored: vitamin deficiency, autoimmune reactions, disturbed lactate-pyruvic ratio, thyroid deficiency, hypothalamic and adrenocortical disturbance, deficient eye-tracking movements, and childhood tonelessness, all suggestive of a polygenetic theory.

Through an elaborate method of computer analysis of the EEG of schizophrenics, Giannitropani (1974) demonstrated that the brain activity of these patients differs from that of the normals in very specific ways. One of the differences is in brain activity in the 29-Hz band, which has been found to be associated with attention mechanisms; focusing on this dimension should produce better information on the nature of the deficit in these patients.

We dealt with psychological theories as well: deficient perceptual feedback, deficiencies in information processing, weakened homeostatic control, social drift, and excessive social role expectations. But the scientific papers in psychiatry tended to represent studies of both significant and insignificant problems—with far too many of the latter. Many merely repeat aspects of the original contributions of others. In community psychiatry, especially, conclusions are often drawn in too short a period of time and without adequate systems of evaluation, and the number of subjects observed and described is far too small.

Many biomedical and clinical reports do not accurately define the clinical entities studied but use worn-out designations, such as "endogenous depression," etc. A multidisciplinary approach to etiology must be based on common definitions and terminology even though systems of ratings and classifications are constantly subject to modification. Statistical data should be based on modern sophisticated analyses, rather than on simple correlations. Too few investigators are trained in the use of a general systems approach.

The future of psychiatry obviously depends on the development of research. However, increased knowledge can only be achieved through increased refinement of research designs and theoretical concepts. The superficial correlations that have satisfied us heretofore are no longer acceptable. Indeed, there are so many complexities to deal with in the study of human personality that young persons interested in investigative careers are often discouraged when they contemplate the intricacies of working in the field of human mentation and behavior. The high degree of variability and the tremendous difficulties in holding parameters constant produce almost intolerable frustration.

The old definition of psychiatry focused on clinical phenomena: that is, with prevention, diagnosis, and the treatment of mental disturbances. Although the function of a medical psychiatrist is to treat patients, we find that there is no sound body of knowledge concerning *what kind of treatment, applied to what kind of patients, by what kind of a person, under what kind of circumstances achieves what kind of results.* It is surprising that this void should exist, despite the contention of many so-called schools of psychiatry that they achieve unsurpassed results in treatment. One cannot deny that contact with a member of the so-called helping professions may bring about some favorable results, but it is by no means clear what actually causes the results that satisfy the therapist. Perhaps a favorable therapeutic outcome may be attributed to contact with an understanding, empathetic human being for variable periods of time, with opportunities for ventilation of feelings and tensions rather than for explanation and interpretation on the part of the therapist.

A newer concept of psychiatry is that it is a conglomeration of contributory sciences—it is obviously predicated on the expectation that advances in psychiatry depend on advances in those sciences. According to this definition, scientific psychiatry, as it should be called, requires an understanding of each of its various parts, unlike the empirical, impressionistic, prejudged, and bias-loaded approach of the past.

If the vast area that today's psychiatry covers is analyzed—and who can guess how much further it will extend?—we find divisions that are based on a number of points of view or orientations. Those concerned with age may deal with children, adolescents, adults, and the aged. Problem-oriented frames of reference may be organized around disease classifications, behavioral manifestations, and dynamic or psychoanalytic concepts. Action-oriented psychiatry is concerned with the study of epidemiology and social engineering, which are primarily dedicated to changing a society, so that the frustrations and conflicts that end in sickness are alleviated. Finally, there is the approach-oriented point of view, which focuses on the biological, psychological, or social aspects of behavior. Sometimes these are linked together in one biopsychosocial approach, and one day perhaps they will be understood as a general system.

The inevitable conflicts that can arise because of this multiplicity of approaches cannot be resolved through a reductionistic or a humanistic frame of reference. General systems theory encompasses several more limited subtheories, each of which may contribute to hypotheses that require well-designed operational research.

The past several decades have seen many significant psychiatric breakthroughs. In its heyday in this country, psychoanalysis was considered to be the answer to all of the problems of mankind. As a humanistic theory concerned with meanings, however, it failed to qualify as a true science. There is no question that some aspects of psychoanalytic theory are extremely fruitful and would be valuable if they were subjected to operational research. I can think of no more important theoretical formulation applicable to clinical psychiatry than the theory of ego-functions, which can be made operational since *ego-functions expressed in behavior are the final common pathways of a wide variety of internal processes.* They must, however, be related to known situations or environmental conditions and studied transactionally.

A psychosomatic breakthrough created optimism that we would find the emotional components of physical diseases and that the specificity so defined would enable us to pinpoint the causes of specific chronic degenerative diseases. Unfortunately, this has not proven to be true. We are finding that there is greater evidence for response specificity than for stimulus specificity. Nevertheless, the psychosomatic concept of differentiation points to the need for a full investigation of the personality types involved either in the cause, course, or results of specific chronic diseases. There is a great deal of work being done, not necessarily entirely psychological, but of importance in determining differences among people who suffer from chronic degenerative diseases.

The discovery of psychotherapeutic drugs, of course, has been a breakthrough of monumental dimensions. Their importance is due not only to their ability to decrease activity, excitement, and anxiety and to alleviate depression, but also to their role in stimulating the study of the specific biochemistry of brain functions in various areas. The paradigm that is being developed leads us to believe that many portions of the brain with discrete functions contributing to the mosaic of behavior may have specific chemical constituents that when they become disordered, may respond to specific therapeutic agents. I look forward to great accomplishment in this field of neuropharmacology.

The concept of prevention leads inevitably to social psychiatry, which is action oriented. It is evident that through a shift in community functions, societies can be developed in which frustration, conflict, and aggression are lessened and mental illness is thereby prevented. Such a pious hope should not be confused with community psychiatry, which is actually a delivery system that organizes medical care.

Since social psychiatry has not yet developed a paradigm, has not yet constructed research designs, and has not yet conceived of techniques for evaluation, it is too early to tell whether or not this field will be productive. I do believe, however, that the role of psychiatry in the *prevention of mental illness* is only secondary. It is the sociologists, anthropologists, and the epidemiologists who will have the primary responsibility for action in this field, using psychiatrists as consultants to set limits on wild social theories.

There is some hope that the study of evoked potentials and other electroencephalographic (EEG) phenomena will develop some discriminatory analyses of behavioral functions, and that the immunological aspects of disease will one day be applied to certain disturbances in the central nervous system. Certainly, the studies of sleep, dreams, and also hypnosis are likely to contribute a great deal to the phenomena of aberrant kinds of thinking and behavior in the psychoses. Another area in which there is a good deal yet to be done is the study of biogenetics. Sound research in child development is still in its early phases (Murphy, 1962). We need to know a great deal about the development of normality in children, adolescents, and adults and the conditions under which ego-functions, particularly in terms of their coping devices, are derived.

Through the *Archives of General Psychiatry,* I have witnessed many changes in psychiatry, but whether they can be labeled progress or not will be determined only by posterity. My hope is that the *Archives of General Psychiatry* will always remain an open forum for new ideas and a source of leadership for the better understanding of man's troubles in a dangerous world (Grinker, 1969b).

The annual reports that I prepared during my years as director of P & PI provide a virtual history of a changing and developing institution and the professional and social milieu in which it has functioned. The introduction to the report of 1963 was a particularly salient summary of the state of psychiatry fifteen years ago, and it would be helpful to quote from it now. It should help us to gauge where we have come since then and where we are going. The assessment of the problems facing the psychiatric institute of the 1960s seems to be a measuring stick against which the issues of education and training facing psychiatry can be evaluated today.

> It seems incredible that only seventeen years ago the United States experienced the beginning of a serious effort to increase the number of psychiatrists needed for a large number of functions that were never carried on before the war. Suddenly, numerous individual hospitals and university departments that had been occupied with the training of one or two psychiatric residents by means of preceptors and on-the-job training expanded their programs to include a large number of residents. This developed as a sequel to the excitement during the war when the possibility of turning out psychiatrists for specific purposes proved successful.
>
> The so-called thirty- or ninety-day "wonders" did an extraordinarily good job in treating the war neuroses, which were an aftermath of the stresses of combat and military conditions. This excitement not only influenced the psychiatrists responsible for conducting departments and institutes and developing training programs, but also the young medical officers who had come into contact with the psychiatric point of view in their approach to psychosomatic problems resulting from stress conditions. Large numbers of these young men, only some of whom had had special courses, became interested in the field and applied for training as psychiatrists. Some even abandoned their partial training in other specialties. Because of their war experiences, they were older and more mature in worldly matters, were more interested in what psychiatry had to offer, and were more prepared to receive it.
>
> Our own experience encompassed the rapid expansion of a prewar residency program, consisting of two trainees, to a postwar program of ten medical graduates who had served during the war as medical officers. These ten constituted a single class, receiving instruction through courses, seminars, conferences, and supervised work with patients. This was our first and only attempt at carrying a group of people together through the entire three years of training without the use of a staggered, graded curriculum developed for classes entering the program each year.
>
> As a result of this preliminary three-year experience, we were better able to plan a graded curriculum in which a certain number of

residents were inducted each year. In fact, our hospital was one of the pioneers in developing a graded curriculum, in setting high standards for selection of residents, and in emphasizing personal supervision in teaching. At first, this program was under the auspices of the Veterans Administration, and only later did we transfer to the NIMH program supported by the United States Public Health Service.

Meanwhile, other similar programs were established throughout the country. The national trend, stimulated and supported largely by the NIMH, was to develop a body of psychiatrists available to treat not only ex-servicemen but the population at large. Gradually, over the years, the numbers of these training programs increased. It is to the credit of the directors of the program and the individuals in charge of the NIMH training branch that the standards of training quickly became universally high, so that the current training programs differ only in some degree of specialization, in the reputation of some of the teachers, and in their geographical location.

Although war experiences, which were so salutary, did not include actual psychoanalytic techniques, our work and teaching were largely based on psychoanalytic theory, which has since that day been called by the euphemism *psychodynamic theory*. As a result, our students entered the specialty of psychiatry with the intention of becoming analysts. These two fields were so interlocked in our own minds that originally we chose our psychiatric residents simultaneously with our local analytic institute. A resident entering training therefore was a candidate for psychoanalytic training. In those days, we turned out people who we hoped were general psychiatrists, but who became analysts and restricted their private activities, as most analysts do, to the office practice of psychoanalysis. However, most of them also remained on our staff as teachers supervising residents' psychotherapy in a one-to-one relationship. As a result, the pedagogical point of view not only maintained its psychodynamic purity but increased in intensity almost to the exclusion of other forms of treatment. Like so many other institutions, we became recognized as proponents of psychoanalytic psychiatry.

Since the beginning of the new kind of residency; programs that quickly multiplied throughout the country, many changes have occurred in the field of psychiatry. It has moved into many new areas. Some seem far distant from psychiatry when it is viewed as a strictly medical specialty devoted to the diagnosis, prevention, and treatment of mental illness.

Some of the extensions of psychiatry have been acclaimed before proof of their validity has even been attempted. Some seem a natural outgrowth of liaison with sciences, such as biochemistry and the social sciences. At any rate, the need to extend our training programs to make general psychiatrists aware of the many factors involved in the causes, course, result, and therapy of the various psychiatric entities was emphasized at a meeting of training psychiatrists sponsored by the American Psychiatric Association in Washington, D.C., in 1962.

It became obvious then that we would have to cram a tremendous amount of information into three years or lengthen the training program to at least five years. The resident, at least during training, obtains a broad general knowledge, later venturing into postgraduate fields for specialization in psychoanalysis or child, administrative, group, family, and social psychiatry, etc., after his residency. All of these, however, require a basic general training.

Now I should like to review briefly some of the problems at every training institute for which solutions must be found.

First, the staff model becomes important, in that it indicates what kinds of psychiatry are operational and are conducted by those in positions of authority. If enough differing models are available instead of one stereotype (for example, a psychoanalytic psychiatrist), these are antidotes to the restrictive specialization now characteristic of most psychiatric graduates. To develop this model means, of course, recruiting people of various points of view to the staff. Unfortunately, they are not easily available, especially for part- or full-time institutional work, and it has become necessary to develop such a series of variegated specialists to serve as models.

The second great problem is *preselection,* which, strangely, is a powerful obstruction to the development of general psychiatrists. The preselection occurs in medical school or as early as college. It occurs because the young aspirant has been unrealistically imbued with the miracle of psychoanalytic psychiatry in cure and reconstruction of personality. The number of individuals who come into the training programs who have not either explicitly, or implicitly, decided on psychoanalytic careers is minimal. When these others appear, their chances for residency are weighted heavily, despite other objections to their appointment. This problem can be solved only by a shift in emphasis during the student's education, in his courses in general psychology and in experiences in medical school.

A third problem is the emphasis in most training institutions on long-term cases supervised continuously by a single teacher with few interruptions and with relative neglect of reevaluation of the patient's progress. For training, we need to select more short-term acute cases that offer a hope of successful adjustment in brief periods of time. We have adopted a policy of changing supervisors every six months, giving each student a maximum of eighteen supervisors during three years of outpatient work, and giving him individual supervisors for each inpatient.

We have recently surveyed our supervisors' seminar and found that its focus of interest is much too narrow, dealing with internal dynamics and psychodynamic processes in therapy. It became necessary to broaden supervisors' educations and to help them experience problems related to matters not involved in the dyadic relationship, such as milieu, family, and group, and to psychopharmacology and other areas extraneous to the usual dynamic formulations of stereotypes.

We have emphasized research conferences that we hold twice a week, once for institutional reports and once for visitors, as well as research activities in which residents participate. A number of distinguished investigators are asked to give lectures at our institute, and they engage in small discussion groups with residents. We now have decided that each resident must complete a piece of research during his three years, and we offer a prize in each class for the best work done.

A number of our staff people are engaged either in full- or part-time research work, and we have a nucleus of full-time basic scientists. Residents are given opportunities to discuss problems, to learn the attitudes of investigators, and hopefully to become inducted into the ranks of clinical investigators, if not into basic science. In an effort to further stimulate this interest, we give a course, in which all investigators in the institute participate, entitled the Biological Foundations of Psychiatry. Our literature seminar takes up the works of distinguished authors, both classic and modern, in an effort to train the residents in critical analysis of published works.

One of the great difficulties in broadening the psychiatric vista of each resident is the highly indigenous language surrounding specific theories. Language actually is not an artificially learned instrument, but represents modes of thinking and conceptual formulations. If one can induce the resident to learn the meanings of the transactional, the sociological, and the communication and informational processes, both conceptually and operationally, he will be able to use the appropriate language for each aspect of modern psychiatry. Since at the present time we have few transformational hypotheses and must view each conceptual system independently or translate one into another by substituting words, it is difficult to achieve a thorough understanding of theoretical differences.

Is our goal in broadening the curriculum for psychiatric residents to create more specialists in part of the extensive field of psychiatry? If this were true, specific training centers could specialize in teaching psychiatric subspecialties. All residents, no matter what branch of psychiatry they eventually select, need a general overview of the field. A knowledge of the total field, the recognized foci of interest within the field, and the transactional processes among those foci is necessary for an adequate knowledge, as well as therapeutic efficiency in any branch selected. A thorough knowledge of the transactional approach may effectively counteract the restrictions competing "schools" may attempt to impose on the graduate student after his residency.

Actually, one of the biggest problems is the student's need for security and certainty and his wish to participate in a field where specific, often dogmatic, statements can be made regarding what is known and what should be done. This need is met in the field of psychiatry only by rigid formulations and the stereotypes that unscientific practitioners promulgate. We try to challenge, to question, to suggest tests, and to indicate alternative hypotheses in order to make the student aware that there are other aspects of psychiatry besides psychodynamics and that there are other frames of reference than the psychoanalytic.

We have a hard struggle ahead of us, and this struggle will last for a long time. Nevertheless, one reassuring note is the fact that although most of the university professors of psychiatry and the directors of the institutes of psychiatric training are psychoanalytically trained (since they are given precedence over those who are not), most of them behave as we do. After a short time, those accredited and senior analysts who accepted positions as directors of training in general psychiatry become transformed. They assume responsibility for the training of general psychiatrists and not psychoanalysts. They are quite permissive in teaching psychoanalytic principles and in the pursuance of psychoanalysis in a postgraduate training program, but they, as we, are struggling to become as broad, as diversified, as objective, and as eclectic as possible.

CHAPTER 5

Definition, Diagnosis, and Classification

Definition is a necessary prelude for the development of science. It embodies the simplistic notion that naming is knowing, or vice versa. Unfortunately, if scientific disciplines were rated according to their exactness and their degree of acceptance, psychiatry would be extremely low in the hierarchy. Definitions are hardly subject to consensus.

Psychiatry has been defined first as a specialty concerned with the prevention, diagnosis, and treatment of mental and emotional disorders. Yet, each of these three functions can be variously interpreted.

Second the definition of a psychiatrist as a physician whose specialty monopolizes these functions no longer holds, because the identical activities engage social workers, psychologists, psychiatric nurses, and even lay persons who have had no professional training. Finally, the definition of mental and emotional disorders as *dis*-eases of the mind has been disputed by mythologists, who believe that such illnesses are only problems of living and are merely labeled as illnesses by psychiatrists for their own nefarious purposes.

To discuss psychiatric problems as universal problems of everyday living does not allow them to fall within the value systems of scientific orientation. Such an approach bypasses decisions regarding specific methods of treatment, which are increasingly dependent on diagnosis. It deprives the professional of the opportunity to prognosticate the future, difficult though that may be. It encourages uniform attitudes and decries the particular contribution that can be made by the trained physician.

To malign psychiatry in such a way is to inhibit its attempts to treat the sick, to prevent suicide and homicide, and to disguise the valiant efforts of the majority of psychiatrists who do their best within the current state of knowledge and available funds. During the two world wars, for example, soldiers suffering from mental illness were often said to be victims of "shell shock," even though they had never heard a gun fired; or of "operational fatigue" or "combat fatigue," although they had not been near the battle front. Such euphemisms only delayed the mentally ill from obtaining proper treatment. To avoid the so-called pejorative psychiatric labels of diagnosis by the use of terms such as "problems of living," which are universal, is to abrogate what help a psychiatrist can give.

The deluge of recent accusations that mental illness is a myth are written and spoken in unscientific, intemperate language destined to appeal to far-right political sectors of the population. Though such accusations are not responsible for psychiatry's weak diagnostic approaches, it is essential that they be responded to, though without the intention of elevating a "myth" to a position worthy of debate.

It is not surprising that psychiatrists are bewildered by professional confusion. They are exposed to rapid changes in their field, and furthermore, they resent and detest governmental regulations regarding kinds of treatment, length of treatment, and resistance of third-party payers. They are deeply upset by adverse public opinion and by the negative coverage the media give their earnest efforts.

Diagnosis in psychiatry has long been neglected, essentially because there are few answers to the questions of "how" (the disease's etiology) and "why" (its teleology or adaptive purpose). Illness is not a rational choice based on decision. Unconscious motivation has long been an accepted principle. It is essential to define the *what* of mental illness in suitable terms—and as accurately as possible.

When Kraepelin and his predecessors established diagnostic criteria in the late 1800s, it was assumed that course and outcome would be specific and that the organic bases for the major psychoses would be found in specific neuronal changes in the brain, but these could not be established or maintained. Without biological and social etiological boundaries, but with the advent of psychoanalysis, clinicians became distinterested in diagnosis, maintaining that their main interest was in the treatment of specific patients and that the diagnosis of the disease and the discovery of its adaptive purpose were unimportant.

The diagnostic dilemma has troubled psychiatrists for more than a century, although the shifts have had differing sequences. The history of psychiatry presented by Alexander and Selesnick (1966) clearly indicates how feelings and attitudes toward the deviances of behavior and their treatments reflect the value systems and ethics of the contemporary culture. There was little advancement in classification and diagnoses before Morel described dementia praecox in 1850 or Kraepelin attempted the total classification of mental disorders in 1883 (translated in 1912). Yet, the latter survived a number of aemendations until after World War II, when a group of military psychiatrists under the leadership of William Menninger revised, but did not essentially alter, the nosological classification.

Before the zenith of Freudian psychiatry, the major emphasis on diagnosis was stimulated by the legalities associated with commitment procedures and the failure of a wide variety of neurological other than "moral" therapeutic approaches to the psychoses. When dynamic psychiatry took hold in the United States, and with the development of ego psychology, emphasis shifted to the understanding of individual patients and their problems, with a corresponding neglect of scientific psychiatry as represented by diagnosis and classification. In his paper, "Psychoanalysis and Developmental Psychology," Heinz Hartmann (1964) gives expression to the revolutionary view that "we come to the conclusion that psychoanalytic psychology is not limited to what can be gained through the use of the psychoanalytic method."

Hartmann (1964) elaborates further on this when he discusses the developmental studies, which "will of necessity lead to a growing awareness of the sign- or signal-function behaviour details may have for the observer, that is, to a better or more systematic understanding of how data of direct observation can be used as indicators of structurally central and partly unconscious developments—in a sense that by far transcends the possibilities of sign interpretation accessible to the various methods of testing."

It is not surprising that diagnostic skill has neither been taught nor regarded as highly significant in psychoanalytic work (A. Freud, 1976). Paul Meehl, (1959), a distinguished psychologist, critically states: "Rather than decrying nosology, we should become masters of it, recognizing that some of our psychiatric colleagues have in recent times become careless and even unskilled in the art of formal diagnosis."

The philosopher Kaplan (1964) indicates that every *classification* discloses relationships that must always be taken into account.

Karl Menninger (1962), in *The Vital Balance* has attempted to resist classification of mental disorders, stating that perhaps there is only one class of mental illness—namely, mental illness. He does, however, indicate the danger implicit in simplification and reduction. Also, he is unable to avoid advancing his own classification, comprising *five levels of adaptive retreat* to maintain equilibrium in the face of emergencies. His five orders of *dysfunction* or *dyscontrol* are stages in the defense against aggressive impulses, which represent in themselves dissolution and are tragic in their outcome. The most informative aspect of this book is the historical account of psychiatric classification from 2600 B.C. to the current development of the *Diagnostic and Statistical Manual* (DSM III).*

Spitzer and Sheehy (1976) state that classification should be an aid in planning effective treatment and predicting likely outcome. They cite the current criticisms: that the DSM III is antihumanistic, that it abandons the legacy of Freud, or that it is too radical. The American Psychiatric Association Task Force on Nomenclature and Statistics, under the chairmanship of Robert L. Spitzer, has worked hard for several years to prepare DSM III. The operational criteria have been difficult for them to establish, because consensus has been difficult to reach. Even psychiatrists are resistant to change.

In psychiatry, diagnosis is not so simple as listening to the

*I was a member of the committee to develop DSM I, but we dissolved when we learned that we were bound by treaty to the internatonal classification. The current DSM III is evoking considerable controversy and discussion and publication will be long delayed.

heart beat and identifying the inefficient valve. As in most clinics, the first attempt at diagnosis is made by the social worker, who screens for admission; then, the resident writes the history, which is discussed at a diagnostic conference. Later, when the patient begins his therapeutic alliance with an assigned therapist, a different diagnosis may be apparent. Finally, after a long-term follow-up, the diagnosis may again seem different. The process of making a diagnosis ends only when and if a firmly determined etiological component outside the psychiatric system is discovered and validation is apparently assured. Even then, variations in the strengths of the etiological factors changing the range of integrations may influence or change the diagnosis. Sound diagnoses must be based on continuing, perceptive clinical judgment.

> We are impressed by the amount of energy that has been expended in both attacking and defending various contemporary systems of classification. We believe that a classificatory system should include any behavior or phenomenon that appears promising in terms of its significant correlates. At this stage of our investigations, the system employed should be an open and expanding one, not one which is closed and defended on conceptual grounds. Systems of classification must be treated as tools for further discovery, not as bases for polemic disputation. [Katz, 1967]

The clinical psychiatrist uses three methods with which to make his diagnosis: observation of accurately described behaviors; interviews, usually in dyadic settings or information from informed sources, usually other members of the patient's family; and psychological test performances.

My own research designs have emphasized a different approach: Instead of using the data of dyadic introspection drawn from interviews, various forms of psychotherapy, or historical or anamnestic data, I describe objective, observable behaviors. Thus, in essence, I observe and describe predominate modes of behaviors and then rate traits extracted from an ego-psychology framework.

In a recent monograph, *The Borderline Patient,* Werble, Drye, and I (1977) have reported in detail a number of current patient protocols. We have underlined the "essence" of the syndrome, recognizing that many more symptoms are present as defenses or substitutes. For example, the borderline, lonely because he gets little satisfaction from interpersonal contacts (object-relations) (Fromm-Reichman, 1950), may instead substitute alcohol, drugs, or homosexuality. These, of course, are not specifically characteristic of the borderline; syndromes are always "mixed." (For a philosophical discussion, see Myuskonic, 1977.)

Several cautions need to be voiced regarding diagnosis. First, recent cases with specific protocols should be used, instead of histories written by students in eras past (the Iowa 500). Second, group familiarity with the words and concepts used is essential. Third, follow-up for evaluation and prognosis is critical. Fourth, fashionable diagnoses of the day must be recognized as likely biases. Studies of the various treatments for mentally ill patients require the establishing of diagnostic categories, defining the methods applicable to each, and developing criteria for results.

The results of earlier attempts at delineation of types of mental illness and the long list of various classifications that have been adopted are no longer adequate, but we must keep trying. Schizophrenia is an example: (1) Many schizophrenics seem to have elevated, excited moods resembling mania. Others are depressed and suicidal, although this mood should be discriminated from anhedonia. We hedge on their label, diagnosing them as neither schizophrenic nor manic-depressive, but as *schizoaffective*. There is no evidence from the clinical data that the thought disorders of both groups are identical. However, about 20 percent of manic-depressives do have some form of thought disorder, though in my opinion, it is quite different from that of the schizophrenic. The notion that these in fact constitute one disease creeps up frequently, but it is not well founded. (2) There is also an attempt to designate the acute schizophrenic, with one or several psychotic breakdowns, as suffering from a disease different from that of the slowly progressive chronic schizophrenic. Such a designation implies what may be called a *schizophrenic spectrum* in the families of index subjects, which may not be found in those of the acute schizophrenics.

The recognition and identification of a schizophrenic spectrum is an important issue in current research. We cannot write about neurotic or psychopathological traits in families or siblings of index subjects because such terms are loosely used and may apply to everyone, and specific syndromes require identification instead of resort to the fragile omnibus of "sick families." Yet, the supposed absence of spectrum diagnoses for relatives of acute schizophrenic index cases is not an indication that the acute are genetically unrelated to the other types. Clinicians know that one or several acute breakdowns may precede the development of a chronic and often irreversible course. The fate of acute schizophrenics can only be determined by a long-term follow-up continuing past age forty. (3) The third issue is the *changing manifestations* of all psychiatric disorders: conversion hysteria, mania, catatonia, and hebephrenia, etc. It is clear that today we see more restricted and constricted characters.

In general, scientific information is obtained by collecting observations and measurements under specific conditions, encoding the data in terms characteristic of the statistical model to be used, processing the data, and checking the results again against the original events. Royce (1964) outlines the standards applicable to clinical research: (1) sufficient opportunities for observations, as on a nursing unit; (2) specified conditions, even though the variables are not controlled; (3) the involvement of persons; (4) observing specified variables; (5) repetitive observations; (6) making statistical analyses leading to the determination of the contribution of each variable. To this we must add (7) the checking of results for their logical relationship with clinical experience.

Referral of patients to clinical psychologists for testing when the diagnosis is uncertain has decreased in the last decade. Although psychometrics, including the Rorschach and TAT, add considerable content, they constitute a framework in which the psychologist is essentially conducting a *clinical interview* not much different from that of the psychiatrist and with far less skill in differentiating common human qualities from psychopathology.

In our quest for certainty, however, we have almost automatically forced natural phenomena and the laws pertaining to them into the strait-jacket of continuity. We tend to close the arc of open circles and demand universal laws because of our abhorrence of discontinuities, belying our empirical information and causing our concepts to become comfortably uniform. This may be one of the reasons why some psychiatrists obliterate obvious differences and try to force all psychopathology into one disease.

How can psychiatric illness be classified? Certainly it is not categorized by means of symptoms (more easily by syndromes) and not by isolated etiological factors that exclude all others (Kaplan, 1964). Ideally, diagnoses can only be made after an exhaustive search for all possible contributing etiological factors. Such a quest tries our patience because it requires too much time and expense and also delays the scientific purposes of diagnostic classification: to enable a wide variety of disciplines to study the "what;" to test a wide variety of treatments, including a natural, spontaneous course; and to determine the life history to the final end. In the meantime, we should abstain from diagnostic nihilism, grand holistic generalizations, and minute classifications.

What we can state, for example, when the schizophrenic organization weakens or breaks is that there are two classes of symptoms, as originally formulated by Hughlings Jackson (1925). One is the loss of functional control determined by the absence of high-level thinking and feeling. These weak or deficient parts often cannot be compensated for by other functions. The other is the presence of old functions, always alive but repressed or controlled, revived by the absence or weakness of regulation.

Another diagnostic issue concerns the adaptive or so-called restitutive functions attempting to cover up the lost or revived functions of the past process. Adaptation is often successful, and possibly no further difficulties will ensue. A short-term outcome, however, is not definitive.

I cannot conclude this chapter on an optimistic note. Definitions are vague, diagnoses are variable, and classifications are insecure. Diagnoses are confused by biases, differences in clinical interviews, and the need for a sound empirical psychiatry. Certainly many possible classifications are dependent on inferences regarding etiology. The crudest classification includes types of neuroses, personality disorders, and kinds of major psychoses.

The unpopularity of diagnosis and the lack of recognition of the importance of the life history of describable entities stem from the reaction to the "disease" concept of mental illness and the overemphasis on "the problem" of the patient and his individual dynamic processes. Syndromes and accurate diagnostic criteria are frowned upon as superficial.

As the final common pathway of inner feelings behavior can serve as a highly accurate index of ego-functions. Child analysts use this approach. Behavior manifests functions ascribed to a hypothetical ego. These are the filtering of perceptions; the expression of motivations, affects, defenses, and compromises; the employment of symptoms and sublimations; and the demonstration of integrative capacities and disintegrative trends.

The "core research operation" must entail: (1) *observing* myriad, diverse behaviors of a large patient sample with a seemingly common ailment and those of samples with different problems; (2) *describing* accurately behaviors frequently repeated (by one person) and replicated (by many persons) ; (3) *classifying* behaviors into "factors"—minute ego categories—and further classifying them into "clusters" of factors; (4) *quantifying* the carefully labeled behaviors by determining their frequency through protracted recording of observations; and (5) *validating* their significance by statistical analysis.

The behavior statistically deemed significant for the general mental category under study is then statistically related to subcategories. From here, etiologic exploration begins.

Anna Freud (1976) warns that this constitutes *only* a beginning, however: "Even supposing that we have complete knowledge of the etiological factors that decide a given result, nevertheless what we know about them is only their quality, not their relative strengths. Some of them are suppressed by others because they are too weak and they therefore do not affect the final result. But we never know beforehand which of the determining factors will prove the weaker or the stronger."

Unfortunately, our systems of diagnosis and classification have been confused by dichotomies. During the last several decades, clinical psychiatric research has become much more sophisticated through the use of detailed, especially constructed interviews; observations of behavior; questionnaires; psychological tests; and follow-back or follow-up studies put together by appropriate rating scales and computer analyses. Improved statistical techniques, such as cluster, discriminate, and principal component analyses and factoring have successfully dealt with quantitative scales in a way vastly more productive than simple scanning or one-to-one correlations.

Yet, psychiatrists have not overcome their anachronistic concepts of dichotomies based on the kind of yes-or-no or night-or-day thinking more appropriate to digital computers than to clinical explorations. We still read and hear of medical versus social models of the mind, of nature versus nurture, of reductionism versus humanism in psychiatry. Indeed, even complementarity, for example, heavy biogenetic preparation requiring low degrees of stress and weak hereditary factors requiring high degrees of stress to produce overt disease, has not completely superseded the concept of single causes in linear effects.

Many protests have been made against dichotomies, against the ignorance by medicine of psychological factors, and against using reductionistic concepts of biochemical levels of dysfunction as the only indicators of disease, making brain dysfunction a problem for neurologists. Problems of living require constant reeducation not easily available to medical men or psychiatrists. Too often, the professionals seem to be going over and over the same ground, with little interchange and cross-fertilization and little educational impact on the wider medical and lay communities.

Distortions may develop not only in definition but in the exclusion of significant data, even by pure clinicians. The dynamic school overlooks much of behavior, and the behaviorally oriented clinician ignores large amounts of data about feelings and concerns. Both have a tendency to overlook biogenetic, family, communication, biochemical, and physiological systems of data that are becoming increasingly understood. Psychodiagnoses in one- or two-hour sessions may be brilliant narcissistic exercises through which the professor can astound his students, but it is known the results are not impressive over the long run. Criticisms of diagnostic reliability and hence usefulness, however, should not result in an abandonment of the process, but should lead to the inclusion of extended areas of information requiring much more time than an interview and/or conference.

Diagnosis and classification are the first steps toward a scientific psychiatry. Despite dedicated therapeutic approaches to individual patients, they must be articulated first within the vocabulary of a traditional clinical framework. It matters not at all, at least to me, whether the labels applied are *disease, disorder, deviance, faulty behavior:* Diagnosis has become a necessity for progress for every aspect of what we call psychiatry.

Only recently have scientific methods been applied in an attempt to understand the rationale, methods, and results of psychotherapy. If we evade the principle that there are categories of mental disturbances, including areas of neuroses, personality disorders, and psychoses, each of which has a specific course and prognosis, then we have no science: There can be no scientific therapy without clinical categories as guidelines to facilitate the study of the life history of specific disturbances, their spontaneous course, and the interrelationships among causative factors.

CHAPTER 6

General Systems and Unified Theories

We have seen that the diagnoses of psychiatric entities, disturbances, or diseases is extremely difficult. Great variations in definition occur within the United States. For example, Texans have a hard time understanding that in the Midwest manic disturbances have decreased, when they see so many. What we (Grinker, Werble, and Drye, 1968) have defined as the *borderline syndrome* appears throughout the United States under a dozen or more labels. Such confusion probably results from the fact that diagnoses are clinical and are not attached to the more defined characteristics derived from other frames of reference.

Clinical diagnoses are based on four important tools. The most important tool is the *interview*. Interviewing a mental patient (whether for diagnosis or research) required much training and experience. It can be done in either a structured or an unstructured manner (I advise a cue sheet for the latter) , in a two-person situation. The second tool *consists of observations of behavior* in a relatively free field (such as a nursing unit, where wide differences between the interview and behavior may be seen. The third technique is essentially an interview within the particular context we call *psychological testing*. Finally, the fourth tool, when feasible, is the questionnaire, which is usually reserved for obtaining follow-up data, and is generally much more effective for the purpose than other techniques.

We often read about the necessity for tests of reliability; but I see little value in them, since multiple observers, testers, or interviewers trained in similar methods, using the same concepts, and the same well-defined words, usually agree closely in their conclusions. Cooperating psychiatrists, or certainly those in some far-distant area, draw observations and conclusions that are often hard to reconcile, but no one would expect anything different. On the other hand, reconciliation of different systematic approaches outside the clinical provides some degree of assurance that the diagnosis has meaning as to etiology, if that variability of syndromes over time is taken into consideration.

The diathesis or susceptibility to specific precipitating factors may be due to minimal brain damage based on prenatal trauma or deprivation or organic brain diseases, a result of early somatic disease. Probably most important are biochemical abnormalities affecting particular functions of the central nervous system. A little-known observation of Escalona and Herder (1959) that infants destined for later troubles are those who react intensely to changes in their environment. Finally, many individuals are anhedonic as children, as if some disturbances in their pleasure centers prevent healthy organization of their affective functions, a deficit likely leading to later mental disorders.

Other early experiences seem to have a profound and prolonged effect on the developing child. Early experiences affect character and personality. The infant may even die from neglectful contact, separation from the family, or death of a parent. The latter may even produce difficulties at a later anniversary date. These are diseases of nonattachment, according to Fraiberg et al. (1975). A baby deprived of human partners as a baby is in deadly peril.

Robbed of his humanity, the baby becomes an adult with a social breakdown syndrome who frequently confirms Dunham's (1971) drift hypothesis.

The amount of descriptive effort required before etiological factors are likely to be discovered has been underestimated, and the pursuit of etiology should represent an end point rather than a beginning for classificatory systems. The process of moving from an empirical to an etiological orientation is, of necessity, inferential and therefore susceptible to the myriad dangers of premature inference. We propose that the greatest safeguard against such prematurity is not to be found in the scrapping of an empirical descriptive approach, but in an accelerated program of empirical research. What is needed at this time is a systematic, empirical attack on the problem of mental disorders. Inherent in this program is the employment of symptoms, broadly defined as meaningful and discernible behaviors, as the basis of a classificatory system. Rather than an abstract search for etiologies, it currently appears more fruitful to investigate such empirical correlates of symptomatology as reactions to specific forms of treatment, outcome in the disorders, and case history phenomena.

The pervasive concern with etiology may derive from a belief that if this were known, prevention would shortly be forthcoming, thus making the present complex problems of treatment and prognosis inconsequential. Unfortunately, efforts to short-circuit the drudgery involved in establishing an empirically founded psychiatry have not resulted in any major breakthroughs. Etiology is typically the last characteristic of a disorder to be discovered. Consequently, we suggest that the search for etiology be put aside and attempted only when a greater number of the correlates of symptomatic behaviors have been established (Ruesch, 1961).

Before I continue to discuss the modern view of psychiatry, it is advantageous to define communications and information theory.

Ruesch and Bateson (1951) viewed communications as the social matrix of psychiatry because disturbances arise from within the specific framework of society and culture and in turn affect them. People internalize a variety of learned roles that are contained in verbal and nonverbal messages appropriate to particular fields. Disturbed communications constitute an essential part of psychopathology. Bateson (1951) has called communication in which contrary messages are transmitted double bind. Most important are *metacommunications,* implicit commands indicating how to interpret the primary message.

People communicate with each other in the current situation by means of transactions. This is more than one person acting on another. Within a specific system, one person acts on another, who in turn feeds back to the originator. The process is reciprocal and cyclical, with each person attempting to understand the other in a particular situation, with constant efforts to correct misunderstandings and distortions.

Psychiatrists realize that in a sophisticated mode of thinking, behavior is seen as a conglomerate of allocated functions designated and studied by several disciplines. Scientific psychiatrists, as contrasted with therapists, try to put all these together in a meaningful relationship or organization, striving toward establishing a unitary theory. As L.L. Whyte (1948) stated, our aim should be the search for "unity in diversity and for continuity in change," which emphasizes one general form beneath all dualisms.

Control and regulation in open living systems are achieved by means of communication, the transmitting of information within feedback arrangements. This involves many complicated reverberatory cycles, rather than simple linear chains such as these implied in "social development." The living organism is not only reactive to its environment, as a robot reacting passively, but it also actively searches for changing goals, by which it differentiates, grows, learns, and evolves. This proposition contradicts the model of man, in which he supposedly searches for needs and for relaxation of tension from his social environment, and in achieving this, achieves homeostasis. There is more to life than maintenance and survival. In fact, the human capacity for symbolic representation functions as a powerful force for change apart from biological evolution. New symbols are transmitted to other generations by means of language. Thus, symbols are the genes of culture (Emerson, 1954).

As a science, psychiatry cannot rest on clinical foundations alone; these focus on emergent disorders of mentation and behavior. However, a host of variables are antecedent and basic, and these by necessity require the work of an equal number of scientific disciplines. Psychiatry as a science can be called a "conglomerate" composed of parts, such as heredity or genetics; anatomy; physiology or the study of functions of anatomical parts of the brain; biochemistry or the study of circulating substances that are necessary for proper brain functions and, therefore, sound mentation; endocrinology or the study of the glands of internal secretion activated as part of stress responses; anthropology; sociology; and psychology.

These parts, represented by corresponding specific disciplines, have certain basic laws of integration, regulation, and relationships with each other that are isomorphic. In addition, each part or level has its own kinds of control. As a whole, they form a system that encompasses all of man as an animal and as a human in health and disease. To understand such systems, it has been necessary to develop a unified or over-arching theory—a general systems theory.

R.S. Lillie (1945) describes man as a metabolic system, outwardly as an objective physical system in space, inwardly as a subjective thinking, feeling, and willing, center of experience. His nature reveals conservative constancy and novelty or process; thus, he is a psychophysical stable system in an integrative field ready to become conscious when novelty is required.

Correlations among the findings of two or three disciplines have been conducted over many years with only meager results, because the end result is usually a dichotomy. Laura Thompson (1969) has written: "It is now recognized that the local population or community in transaction with the effective ecosystem of which it forms a part, when perceived as a changing event in space-time is one of the most promising units of research for elucidating universal biocultural problems involving human groups."

Wallerstein and Smelser (1969) also link two disciplines—psychoanalysis and sociology—indicating that "psychological and social forces continuously interpenetrate as they impinge on human nature." The theories of both are necessary if we are to develop an adequate theory of man. Such a two-part correlation, interestingly enough, omits the biological—unless the psychoanalytic is somehow considered as biological. But Wallerstein and Smelser also believe that more knowledge will be generated and there will be a greater change in moral values if the two fields of psychoanalysis and sociology are articulated in a complementary fashion.

Some writers indulging in hyperbole have indicated that we are passing through a third "revolution" (They consider classification as the first and psychoanalysis the second). Depending on their special interest, some have designated the development of group therapy, others the development of community psychiatry as the revolutionary trend. Unnoticed by almost everyone, however, there is a slow shift in theory toward consideration of more general, all-encompassing, or unified theories of human behavior. Various terms, such as *holistic, biopsychosocial, general systems theory,* or *unified theory,* have been applied to these global theories.

Weiss (1973) states clearly that the atomistic point of view does not reduce the immense variety of our experiences to a few common denominators. Our basic fallacy is that we have developed as atomists (perhaps he would also say that we have regressed to reductionism). We are trying to atone for our sins and repair the damage we have done by breaking up the universe into units and dealing with them as if they were isolated. We dissect relations among smaller systems and then clumsily attempt to restore them. He adds, "If we had come down from the universe gradually through the hierarchy of systems to the atoms, we would be much better off. Instead we now have to resynthesize the conceptual bonds between these parts which we have cut in the first place."

It is a simple matter to enumerate the various sciences that are, significantly involved in understanding human behavior. These would, in general, include genetics, general biology, anatomy, physiology, biochemistry, pathology, psychology, and all the social sciences. This is a vast array of disciplines, all of which should be recognized as extremely important for some aspect of behavior, although obviously as a group they cannot possibly be mastered by any one person or even by a group of reasonable size.

The number of scientific disciplines involved in the total field of psychiatry seems to represent a vast array of irreconcilable viewpoints. Indeed, each represents an organized way of viewing nature, utilizing special concepts, methods, and evaluations. Each views behavior in a special context, from a specific frame of reference. Such differences should not be minimized, because each system under study possesses processes regulated by somewhat different invariants. Important as these differences may be, they need not isolate the contributory sciences from each other. One method of relating systems of varying orders of complexity is through the use of analogies. The symbol in the human societal system is analogous with the gene in the genetic system; psychologically, learning is analogous with physical growth. Homeostatic mechanisms and variability may be analogized as a similar process from cell to society; part-whole relationships are certainly capable of being viewed as analogous throughout all systems. Analogizing, however, is only a useful preliminary method; although satisfying, it adds little to knowledge of relationships among systems. Translating concepts from one living or life-derived system to another (biologizing psychology or psychologizing sociology) is tautologous rather than unifying. What is needed is a unified theory.

Of the so-called global theories, the one initially stated and defined Bertalanffy (1966-1968) under the title of *general systems theory* has taken the strongest hold. At that time, he attempted to counteract the still-current concepts that an organism is a summation of its parts, by proposing that systems were wholes in themselves, although volumes of writings had previously affirmed this concept. They have attributes of primary action instead of reaction; are dynamic instead of static; and develop by progressive differentiation.

The greatest value of a theory lies in its suitability for the testing of derived hypotheses. Such heuristic values may not be apparent at first. General systems theories enable the investigator to have confidence that there are some natural laws of insomorphism and insofunctionalism and that research can discover both one's position as an observer with respect to evolution, birth, growth, stability, and death, as well as their effects on the observed. The theory enables us to wander through forests of the unknown with some confidence that there are pathways to be found.

Global theories are usually not operational. However, when they are umbrellas encompassing subordinate theories that are closer to empirical or experimental and experiential data, that interact but are not necessarily representative of the same frame of reference, they are extraordinarily fruitful. Thus, for example, some of the subordinate or atomistic theories involved in the general systems concept include part-whole relationships and gradients. They involve concepts of integration and processes of maintaining integration (negative entropy) by means of homeostatis or cybernetic feedback processes and the transmission of information rather than the, physiological concepts of energy. There are subtheories concerned with defenses against disintegration, there are developmental theories concerned with the ontology of activity, and finally, there is the transactional point of view which concerns the interface between sub- and whole systems and between whole systems themselves. Each one of these subtheories can be utilized in relation to the events or activities in nature. Each one of them is dynamic, since they are all concerned with behaviors or actions, rather than with the essence or the naming of parts in a metaphorical sense.

Even so, an encompassing general theory could not have thrived if many less abstract, or let us say "smaller," theories had not been fruitful in stimulating empirical and experimental biological investigations. These were developed by the great naturalists, such as Childs, Coghill, Herrick, and Lillie, etc., who were together at one time at the University of Chicago and who now seem outdated. I was fortunate enough to have all of them as my teachers, but there were others working in their field as well.

Perhaps it would be helpful to enumerate the Chicago group's basic subtheories, recognizing the list is not complete:

1. Living organisms are hypothetical "wholes" characterized by functions which are not simply the sum of its parts but subserve new emergent purposes (Childs, 1941).

2. Within a living organism, control and regulation develops by centralization of function radiating to substructures in a characteristic gradient (Herrick, 1949).

3. An organism matures gradually, or in sudden critical periods makes jump-steps, by means of the differentiation of primary undifferentiated structure-functions (Coghill, 1929).

4. Organisms have the capacity to regulate the input of stimuli from external sources, thereby avoiding constant bombard-

ment, and to maintain their surroundings in a relatively steady state. Their boundary structures are thus semipermeable (Lillie, 1945).

5. The principle of equifinality emphasized by Bertalanffy (1968) is the same as that termed by Hughlings Jackson (1925) *the final common pathway.* Thus, many divergent organic processes may be expressed in ultimate outcome or action through a common structure and thus will result in similar if not identical effects.

6. Living organisms maintain themselves in the face of change within a healthy range of homeostatic processes (Cannon, 1963), or feedback mechanisms. Those in the physical world are termed *cybernetic.* The most successfully studied mechanism is the neuroendocrine system of control and regulation.

7. A living organism is not a self-acting system, and neither in growth nor maintenance can it be torn from the environment with which it forms a so-called system; it is an open system in constant exchange with the physical and living world.

8. Living organisms are open systems of increasing organization from growth through maturity, thereby functioning to increase negative entropy, as contrasted with the physical world of closed systems.

9. Organisms search out for their goals in a purposeful manner to maintain and regulate life. They also are goal-changing, reaching out beyond need gratification, utility, or preservation and thereby becoming creative and evolving (Menaker and Menaker, 1965).

10. Information within and between organisms is not linear (cause and effect or two variable systems) but consists of variable reverberating "circular" transactions establishing complicated chains of causation in which all effects become causes and vice versa. Causality as a goal is superseded by concepts of threshold and by temporal and quantitative properties of a wide number of responses in which the end point may vary by virtue of changing conditions or whose final state may be the end point of a variety of intermediate processes.

These brief statements summarize vast areas of investigation carried out by the great naturalists. It is Bertalanffy's genius that he put them together with the imprint of his own emphasis to speak out against the physicochemical model for biology, psychology, and sociology. Life cannot be explained by reductionistic theories, nor can living, which is an open system-process, be compared with the closed system of the physical world. Rather than reasoning from one system to another by analogy, Bertalanffy attempted to establish living isomorphisms and to develop principles applicable to all living systems at levels from the cell to the whole man. His general system is thus a huge "complex of components in mutual interaction."

Exciting attempts to develop a unified theory, of which general systems theory seems to be the most inclusive, have become intensified lately and have caught the interest of many psychiatrists. Perhaps only a philosopher of science could explain this sudden current interest. Viewed in the context of the history and evolution of social thought, scientific unified theories are a product of twentieth-century thinking, although their rudiments are to be found throughout the history of self-conscious man. Aside from these age-old concerns about the meaning of life and the purpose of man, the nineteenth-century scientific developments in biology, psychology, and sociology, including psychoanalysis, were the essential foundations and developed the necessary conditions that were needed before concepts of the unity of science could be developed. In this sense, contrary to Weiss's opinions, it is clear that atomistic approaches had to come first. The problem in the twentieth century is to bring the diversity of living systems now subserved by specific disciplines, each communicating with its own scientific jargon about a part of the whole, under the umbrella of a unified theory and related to each other by a bridging dynamic scientific language.

The direct application of unified theory to psychiatry would seem to apply to the diagnosis and theory of wholes larger than the individual, such as the family, groups, and even larger organizations. For example, community psychiatry is dependent on a concept of systems and their transactions. Although we seem to be moving away from the individual with his internal dynamics and psychopathology, if only in terms of, exclusive emphasis, the entire concept of diagnosis and understanding of disease is based on the understanding of how the psyche as a system develops and organizes into a comprehensive whole.

It seems clear that severe stress or strains in later life evoke, in addition to various specific stress responses or defensive maneuvers, partial dedifferentiation, disorganization, or disintegration of system attributes. Then, the total system begins to break down into the parts that have been important in the development of the more organized integrative states. It is then that the various parts reveal in their own way the impact of the earliest experiences which have impinged upon the still undifferentiated organisms. This is the essence of psycho- and sociopathology.

In summary, cognitive and perceptual dysfunctions, for example, in schizophrenia, are on a continuum with those seen in normal persons. They are phasic. There is considerable evidence that the structures for adaptive thinking and perceiving are not obliterated. The stable cognitive control systems that assure adaptation function relatively well under some circumstances. However, these structures are interfered with by a process of disinhibition that disorganizes or interrupts adaptive cognition. The psychological representation of this general disturbance may manifest itself as a disengagement of involuntary attention (Holzman, Levy, and Proctor, 1976). In our institute, not only Holzman's work but also that of the psychophysicist, Koh, revealed the same principle. In Koh's work, attention, and memory in schizophrenia were not independently disturbed, but the integration and synchrony showed a disinhibition that exposed the cognitive disturbances. Thus, in schizophrenia, at least, there is a failure of inhibition, regulation, and control in some superordinate mechanism. The following clinical observations have been made:

1. Failure of inhibitory control is a failure of the organizational function whenever that is localized.

2. The parts under control of this function may substitute for each other, but only the central control may inhibit or be inhibited.

3. There is no question that multiple stimuli, i.e. in the nurs-

ing unit, may result in involuntary lapse in cognitive control in contrast to the eye-to-eye "hold" in two-person interviews.

4. Sudden episodes of confusion are almost always reported to be associated with disturbances in concentration, both involuntary. These lead to anxiety and an increment of disorganization. "How do you reestablish control?" I ask these subjects, who respond with a variety of idiosyncratic attempts. Some just wait it out; others use some interfering activity or different cognitive focusing.

The essential components of general systems theory have been outlined as a metatheory. Many years of resistance were influenced by the fact that psychiatry for a long period of time was only a medical specialty and dominated by psychoanalysis, which had its own umbrella called *metapsychology*. When scientific or research psychiatry became part of the behavioral sciences, a general theory was needed to counteract the parochialism of its contributory sciences.

Tired of senseless controversy about causes, psychiatrists became convinced of multicausality and reciprocal relations, rather than linearity of cause and effect. As a result, the probabilities of the systems approach were enhanced. This did not make it any less possible for a scientist to cover the entire field, but he could feel more comfortable knowing where he was, instead of endlessly riding around in search of boundaries.

Psychiatrists began to recognize that systems and subsystems constituting hierarchies, bounded by permeable borders encasing reverberating transactions, had structure functions and integrative processes. But more than that, they realized that a system functions in relation to other systems. In fact, the proof or validation of a system's functions cannot come from within, but must depend on its "purpose" in relation to another system. This respectable teleology gives a meaning to human research that, admitted or not, is the goal of science; it is certainly not simply a game that we enjoy playing.

CHAPTER 7

Psychosomatic "Medicine": Its Psychiatric Linkages

A CRITICAL ANALYSIS of existing theories and hypothesis becomes necessary from time to time if complacency is to be fought and thinking is to be stimulated. Such an analysis has been long needed in the field of psychosomatic medicine, which, as its name implies, has been concerned with those who are physically sick. Psychosomatic principles have not been well enough formulated, and a coherent body of knowledge has not yet been successfully compiled, nor have operational procedures been adequately developed. Diagnoses are hastily arrived at on the basis of shadowy stereotypes, and rapid or brief methods of therapy are advocated for the most deep-seated and recalcitrant chronic dysfunctions and the most rigid psychological defenses.

The term *psychosomatic* connotes more than a kind of illness: It is a comprehensive approach to the totality of an integrated process of transactions among many systems: somatic, psychic, social, and cultural. It deals with a living process that is born, matures, and develops through differentiation and successive stages of new forms of integration of parts and other wholes. It deals with stresses, strains, and adjustments, with acute emergency mechanisms, disintegrations, and chronic defensive states or disease. In fact, *psychosomatic* refers not to physiology or pathophysiology, not to psychology or psychopathology, but to a concept of process among all living systems and their social and cultural elaborations.

As one considers these transactional processes, it bcomes clear that no further refinement in the biological or social sciences or in the psychological disciplines is necessary to begin the development of sound psychosomatic concepts. Any available, adequate hypothesis in any field and any tool of observation and measurement that can be used by any discipline are suitable to further psychosomatic understanding, providing that the organismic-environmental transactional field is not dichotomized.

Yet, there are many inherent difficulties in carrying out successful psychosomatic research. A stress response to physical stimuli is relatively easy to correlate with the strength of the stimulus; in fact, in experimental pharmacology, the development of dose-response curves is a standard procedure. Psychological stimuli, however, have no standard responses, and attempts to apply graded stimuli in order to evoke graded responses and to determine specific thresholds have been futile.

For a stimulus to have stress-evoked qualities, it must have personal meaning to the subject or constitute a universally appropriate threat. The latter is demonstrated by the fact that strangeness of the experimental room and apparatus even on a preexperimental day is stressful for most subjects, since it violates the human need for rapid cognitive orientation accompanying change. Under these conditions, subjects with low anxiety respond to specific elements in the environment with considerable intensity, whereas those with high anxiety respond less to specific stimuli, but instead experience a gradual decrement of anxiety over time.

We cannot predict with any certainty which personal stimuli may be meaningful to a given subject. For example, during a simple experiment with personnel moving in and out of the experimental chamber on appropriate occasions, it cannot be determined which subjects will respond with anxiety to being alone or to being with people. A knowledge of the personality of the experimental subject and his sensitive conflict areas affords clues to his vulnerability or proneness to specific probing stimuli. Fairly successful predictions can be made as to the nature of the general stress response, i.e. anxiety, anger, or depression. Although quality may be known, the necessary quantity of the stimulus to evoke a response is determined only by trial and error.

Most successful in the production of stress responses are nonspecific stimuli that impugn the subject's perceptual accuracy, threaten psychological disintegration, or impede or block communication. These are much more effective than defense-removing, unconscious conflict-probing specific stimuli, although lately, motion pictures with a known central plot are being used for this purpose. This technique requires careful control, especially concerning prior experiences and adaptations and interpretations of the many possible meanings of the plot. For example, a group of healthy college students did not respond with anxiety on viewing a movie showing a bloody operation because they had, unknown to us, witnessed many gory pictures of lung extirpations shown by a dean who hoped thereby to discourage smoking. Implicit attitudes are also a handicap, in that patients in hospitals or clinics undergoing stress experiments do not readily accept threatening predictions that placebo capsules will make them sick or that physician-experimenters would in any way harm them.

Research on stress is handicapped by the fact that technical difficulties are present under all conditions: In studying stress responses in life situations, in special field conditions such as war or training in dangerous skills, or in experimental and contrived situations. Efforts at teasing out the relative significance of general laws (nomothetic) and the special reactions or events (ideographic) require much greater control over the stimuli employed than heretofore applied. Specificity of stimuli is not a simple matter. Scientific studies require controls that are difficult to achieve in humans with their wide range of perceptions, experiences, and sensitivities. Yet, it is necessary to determine comparable responses or their absence when a stressor is not applied.

Meaningful *psychological* stimuli evoke a variety of defensive psychological responses patterned in the individual and evoking stereotyped emotional and endocrine disturbances, no matter what the stimulus. In fact, such a severe nonspecific stressor as epinephrine, which almost universally stimulates anxiety, is accompanied by physiological and subjective responses characteristic of the subject's stress-evoking experiences in his past life and the situation in which he finds himself.

Since our research designs prohibit action, the emotional responses of anxiety, anger, and depression, or combinations of them, become apparent. These may be observed as behavioral manifestations in gestures, movements, or facial expressions, etc. They are also reportable by the subjects during the experience or are captured by interviews immediately after the experiment. There is a high reliability between observers' rating and self-ratings, both in quality and degree of emotional arousal. It is clear that, to minimize inferences, we cannot work with so-called unconscious affects. Using only verbally or behaviorally reportable emotions may narrow the field of content, but these alone are reliable and achieve validity.

There is another serious problem in psychosomatic research that arises when physiological and psychological responses are disparate. This is the problem of defenses. How and to what degree does a person adapt to or cope with the psychological stress, and how do these defenses influence the homeostatic processes?

Here we have entered a field that requires special methods of observations, interviewing, reporting, and rating. Defenses or protective devices against stress responses may be divided into at least three categories of defenses. In the first, the cues may not be consciously recognized by denial of perception or distortion of reality, so that the significance of the stimulus is not perceived—the "I won't look" technique.

The second group of psychological defenses is directed toward the affect itself, which is difficult for man to endure. For example, anxiety maintains alertness and interferes with sleep and is usually physically and mentally "unpleasure." Man ascribes it to external causes, calls it fear, and moves away from the projected situation or person. Perhaps he sets into operation numerous psychological defenses that become, as rituals, phobias, withdrawals, and regressions, the symptoms of some psychiatric syndromes. Social unrest is also dealt with by the devices of repression.

The third category of defenses is directed against the effects of anxiety. Ego-functions become strained to decrease the difficulties arising from lengthened perception-decision times, inaccuracy, decrease in confidence, and inability to learn. The source of danger becomes generalized and objectless, and discriminatory functions are lost. There is usually an accompanying feeling of disintegration, and this last-ditch defense may actually be a psychotic regressive break.

The highly acclaimed "breakthrough" into the understanding of the course of a variety of degenerative diseases, by ascribing a specific emotional etiology to each, has been disappointing. Psychosomatic research focusing on specific syndromes has been superseded by psychophysiological investigations utilizing modern instrumentation into the phenomena of relationships between mind and body, concentrating mainly on emotions for the mental and on autonomic and endocrine functions for the somatic.

In this chapter's title I have chosen to place quotation marks around the word "medicine," to indicate my reservations about the psychosomatic approach, and the categorical statement made by Alexander when he said, "The attempt to single out certain disease as psychosomatic is erroneous and futile. Every disease is psychosomatic because both psychological and somatic factors have a part in its cause and influence its course. This assumption is valid even for such specific infectious diseases as tuberculosis."

After World War II, many physicians sought training within the newly created specialty of psychosomatic medicine, unaware that *psychosomatic* means a conceptual approach to *relationships* in health *and* sickness, not new physiological or psychological theories of disease or new therapeutic approaches to illness.

At a meeting in New York in 1939, the American Psychosomatic Society and its journal *Psychosomatic Medicine* were founded. I was a charter member of the society and a member of the editorial board until 1977, and I have been able to observe these two enterprises at first hand.

In 1935, Flanders Dunbar had written a pioneering study, *Emotions and Bodily Changes,* in which she developed personality and behavioral profiles of specific diseases. Alexander (1950) used psychoanalytic concepts to elucidate unconscious repressed specific emotions in relation to various psychosomatic diseases. It is interesting to note that the term *psychosomatic* was preceded by hundreds of years in which writers and philosophers (especially the Greeks) were deeply interested in the mind-body problem. Practically every book or chapter on the subject points to a different originator of the field. In my own work, I have cited Henry Holland, who wrote in England in 1852: "Scarcely can we have a morbid affection of body in which some feeling or function of mind is not concurrently engaged directly or indirectly, as cause or as effect."

Yet, the Cartesian dualism, which for many years separated mind as subject and body as object created a dichotomy that even now blocks unitary concepts: For a long time, the German physiologists were the most advanced in the correlation of diseases with the vegetative nervous system. Writers in the twentieth century have suggested that mind and body are two foci of an identical process. It was 1939 before all of these speculations were put together in focus and clear perspective, when a flurry of publications appeared reflecting diverse viewpoints. Still, it was many years before a more general or unified biopsychosocial system was understood and the psychosomatic field was invaded by coteries of basic scientists. Eventually, psychiatrists lost interest in *Psychosomatic Medicine* with its highly technical correlations between biochemistry and physiology, with vague psychological reports relating to about fifteen organs. A new society and journal seemed inevitable, one that would avoid stressing neurological and hormonal mechanisms, autonomic conditioning, and faulty psychophysiological development. A new approach—the social—was to come into fashion.

It is no surprise that the psychosomatic field, which involves both health and disease, has been dominated by psychoanalytic theory through its concepts of psychic energy, i.e. "What cannot be externally expressed in verbal or motoric behavior spends its force internally producing disturbances in organs innervated by the autonomic nervous system, and resulting eventually in tissue changes." Since Freud dismissed the age-old mind-body relationship by his famous phrase, "The mysterious leap from psyche to soma," modern theorists have attempted to find explanation for mechanisms of relationships, while at the same time, speaking of mind-body unity. The psychosomatic field has been dominated by conceptual theories, creating clinical stereotypes based on historical reconstructions, single causes, two variable correlations, and many assumptions and inferences, but few operations have predictive value.

Alexander's psychosomatic research was begun in Berlin and developed further in Chicago with sixty-three papers and books co-authored with his faculty. His concepts involved many uncontrolled variables, complicated research designs, and considerable slippage in reliability. Yet, his ideas became so fashionable that psychiatrists and students could always find in their interviews of patients data that confirmed Alexander's hypotheses about specific psychosomatic disturbances. The fashion continued for many years, even after his migration to his last post in Los Angeles in 1968.

By Alexander's definition, unlike hysterical conversion symptoms, which were assumed to be symbolic expressions of emotional tension, psychosomatic disturbances, in the narrower sense of the word, are vegetative responses associated with chronic emotional states. However, the sharp differentiation between vegetative and somatic systems is not correct. Furthermore, patients laboring under the same emotional conflicts may reveal varying somatic symptoms. Their physiological regressions to more global dedifferentiation occur regardless of the stimulus in a manner specific to their own life patterns.

The journal *Psychosomatic Medicine* was based on the "specificity theory" of Franz Alexander, who contended that each of seven diseases (bronchial asthma, rheumatoid arthritis, ulcerative colitis, essential hypertension, neurodermatitis, thyrotoxicosis, and duodenal peptic ulcer) was aroused by unexpressible specific emotions. Only the vegetative components were present in overfunctional action, leading ultimately to morphological change. For years, the journal was inundated by reports of psychoanalytic investigations confirming this specificity.

Alexander (1950) defined seven conditions and their causes as psychosomatic. These are outlined with their supposed psychogenic components:

1. Bronchial asthma–threatened detachment from the mother.
2. Rheumatoid Arthritis–difficulty with aggressive hostile impulses.
3. Ulcerative colitis–lost hope that tasks involving responsibilities can be accomplished.
4. Essential hypertension–struggle with asserting self.
5. Neurodermatitis–Hunger for love as demonstrated by stroking.
6. Hypothyroidism–fear of biological death.
7. Peptic ulcer–frustration of dependent and oral desires.

The idea that a unique personality type or a specific intrapsychic conflict is essential to the development of a specific disease can no longer be entertained. It was evident that new methods and sophisticated apparatuses had to be used in any effort to establish general relationships between stress stimuli and biological responses. The literature has been flooded with physiological and biochemical researchers that are only weakly related to clinical problems.

My own writing (1954) pointed to greater complexity than Alexander had taken into account:

> As we have briefly summarized investigations into stress-responses, defenses and coping devices in the hope that a better understanding of so-called psychosomatic disorders may result, we have been handicapped by the fact that our experiments can only be conducted on humans in a restricted laboratory space comparable to an animal cage, and for a brief period of time. Such conditions are dissimilar to the free field in which animals roam and humans live, and far short of the time-span needed for the development of human illness. For such an understanding we should know a great deal about the human life-cycle since significant stimuli, stress and coping responses, adaptations, health, and illness vary with phases of the cycle. Just one banal example; the homeostatic range of the child is so wide that the sick child may appear to be dying one hour and completely recovered the next. The aged may give little somatic evidence of serious illness and expire quickly. Certainly the psychosomatic and psychiatric problems vary greatly with phases of the life-cycle.

Today there are few people who (like Alexander) believe exclusively in the linear model–which holds that a psychological conflict *causes* a physical disease. Minuchin (1975) asserts that the overprotective, rigid family provides little opportunity for conflict resolution and uses the field-dependent child as a scapegoat. Mirsky (1968) uses a constitutional plus social stress model for peptic ulcer: Constitutionally increased pepsinogen secretion plus frustrating social events equals the disease. Ruesch 1968 writes about infantile personalities with problems in communication. Neal Miller (1951) uses an operant conditioning model, and with Dunbar (1935) writes about constitution almost exclusively; and Alexander, French, and Pollock (1968) use a psychodynamic model. I early used a field concept. Grace and Graham (1952) consider psychological attitudes most responsible for specific diseases. Spitz (1950) believes early infantile experiences are important for future health.

Definite correlations between psychological and somatic processes now seem simpleminded. It is more productive to enumerate single factors that have been used as explanatory concepts. These include hereditary constitution, birth injuries, organic diseases of infancy that increase the vulnerability of certain organs; the nature of infant care (weaning habits, toilet training, and sleeping arrangements); accidental, physical, traumatic experiences of infancy and childhood; the emotional climate of the family and specific personality traits of parents and siblings; later physical injuries; or later emotional experiences in intimate personal and occupational relations. These factors, in different proportions, are of etiological significance in all diseases. The psychosomatic point of view merely added the psychological factors to those that have long been given exclusive attention in medicine. It is now known that only the consideration of all these categories and their interaction provides a complete etiological picture.

It is interesting that investigators working in the psychosomatic field write and speak loudly of the totality of the whole man, yet limit their work to small segments. There is a vast difference between rigorous biochemical and physiological research and sloppy psychological anecdotes. Certainly psychoanalytic studies are necessarily subjective and stereotyped, and interviews in depth can be used to confirm any desired theoretical point of view. The best we can hope for at this time is to consider the psychosomatic as one mode of approach, but Alexander belies even this when he differentiates between hysterical conversion symptoms and vegetative neuroses, even though both involve somatic and sympathetic nervous systems. As Mirsky (1968) states, there is a large amount of speculation but little data. If all levels of the organism are involved, we need a common language for the totality.

Depending on the focus of interest, we need methods to ascertain the emotional deficiency suffered by infants, the degree of felt separation from the mother, and the temperament of the child as it influences his subsequent behavior. However, readers of the current literature complain that it is either too psychoanalytic or too biological or too social.

It is imperative that we study each system in relation to other systems. Each proposition involves separate operational procedures and different frames of reference. If these can be synthesized, a single building block for a unified theory may be at hand. Such a synthesis would embody the following principles:

1. All functions of the living human organism, whether in health or illness, are psychosomatic.
2. All disturbances in human function are adaptive and involve multiple processes and causes.
3. Varying constellations of processes may find the same functional expression in a final common pathway.
4. The total human organism in varying interrelationships with other organisms and the material world, as well as the individual functions of any single human organisms, are viewed as transactional processes in fields of observer-defined extent.
5. Rather than employing the notion of psychic energy, we must view relationships from the frame of reference of communications and the transmission of information. This is possible whether we are talking about social psychological, or somatic behavior.
6. The influence of strain on the organism differs with the phase of the developmental process or the state of regres-

sion at the time, and that stress is the sum total of organismic response.

7. Heredity, constitution, strength of instinctual forces, life experiences with the first nuclear family and ever-extending social groups, and precipitating factors, etc., are all important in the production of illness. Each has a place in the transacting field of strain and adaptation.
8. The organs that comprise the human body should not be isolated as single targets for a study of healthy function or illness, for they are organized into open systems with highly permeable boundaries.

The idea that unique personality type or a specific intrapsychic conflict is essential to the development of a psychosomatic disease is, I repeat, no longer adequate. Correlations between the physiological and psychological systems have been more important than linear "cause-and-effect" concepts. It is now clear that there is general response to stress stimuli with or without conscious emotional arousal, without differentiation, among the primary affects of anxiety, anger, depression, or pleasure. The general response is largely within the pituitary-adrenocortical axis and suggests a preparatory facilitation of stress responses that are individually specific ("response specificity"), which occur no matter what the stimulus may be (Grinker, 1966b). It may be constitutional, inherited, or acquired early by conditioning experiences. What is psychological, is the subject's appraisal of the meaning (dangerous or not) of stimuli to his comfort, integrity, or very existence, and how he defends himself against false interpretation of these meanings. He does, however, know that, whatever the meaning, he reacts in his personal way, whether this is diarrhea, sweating, tachycardia, or tremor. Our own research (after much time, energy, and work) has shown that a variety of stress stimuli can produce not only general adaptational mechanisms, but also specific responses in individuals. It is on these principles that the theory of response specificity has been developed.

Psychosomatic theory postulates that "given the presence of potentially pathogenic stimulation, conditions would be optimal for the manifestation of disease if there exists a high biologic disposition, the individual's personality structure is such that some change in the psychosocial environment is perceived as 'stressful,' and the individual is unable to cope with the altered environmental circumstances."

In an overview of psychosomatic medicine in the 1970s Lipowski (1977) indicates that the field has made a spectacular comeback. It has become less reductionistic and more holistic and ecological. The relationships have indicated firmer biopsychosocial determinants signified by the words *unified, integrative, holistic,* and *dynamic.* It is now clear that there are no single causes; psychosomatic diseases are especially not exclusively psychogenic or cured by psychotherapy. Although the mediating mechanisms are unknown, the precipitating stimuli cannot be counted; they are social situations that are meaningfully dangerous enough to the subject to evoke, first, a generalized response (from Selye), and then an individually specific local response. They are not, as Engel (1971) states, a part of a specific process of "giving up," but are multicausal.

As Selye (1973, 1976) has recently indicated, to survive, man needs some degree of stress or change. A total resting state is impossible. However, he needs to increase his response to "eustress" and avoid or decrease his reaction of distress, which is the instigator of disease processes.

Without question, psychiatry has many insights to contribute to the understanding and treatment of disease. In an attempt to assure an "input" from our profession, psychiatric consultations have been in use for many years and are still standard practice in many hospitals. Regrettably, however, consultation is solitary, and discussion rarely ensues except over the telephone.

Liaison psychiatry attempts to establish more of an ongoing relationship between the psychiatrist and the medical service. The psychiatrist usually makes rounds with the physicians assigned to a case, becomes well known, and remains a significant part of the medical team. Sometimes the interaction is so gratifying that the psychiatric consultant remains in this role for years, although in services where the death rate is high (as in oncology) or where the psychiatrist may find himself involved in life-and-death decisions (as in the renal dialysis and associated transplant clinic), he may not remain for as long a period of time.

At Michael Reese Hospital we have conducted a wide variety of liaison services over the last thirty years, and consultations, except for emergencies, are conducted during regular business hours. Our positive achievements in terms of service and teaching are exemplified by increasingly more requests for liaison service time. The essential nature of psychiatric education for nonpsychiatric staff, residents, and medical students is becoming more often recognized, and we are confident that it is in such interchange that the frontier of psychosomatic research will one day be expanded.

CHAPTER 8

Coping with Stress and Anxiety

THE PIONEER investigator of the effects of stress on health and disease has been Hans Selye, who began writing about the *general adaptation syndrome* about forty years ago and has continued his studies (1973, 1976). Any stimulus, according to Selye, may serve as a stressor in provoking prolonged generalized adaptations, which in turn become pathogenic for a variety of diseases. Selye raises the questions as to what stimuli can act as stressors, how these phenomena are conducted to the body by the nervous system and the endocrine glands, and what diseases result. His arguments are extremely complicated, and he concedes, "Everybody knows what stress is, but nobody knows what it is" and "Complete freedom from stress is death." Selye's general adaptation syndrome recognizes three stages: (1) alarm, (2) resistance, and (3) exhaustion. The generalized syndrome has been well studied, but the specifics of the alarm and of the responses are still in need of further research.

The problem of *anxiety* occupies a central position in the understanding of psychosomatic and psychiatric processes. Anxiety is conceived to be a basic process in personality functioning, which in the normal, healthy person exists in quantities sufficient to maintain alertness, to anticipate danger by apprehension, and to facilitate mental functioning. In greater quantities, however, anxiety, disrupts ego-functions and controls, partially causes regression of differentiated somatic and psychological functions to more primitive states, and disrupts interpersonal relations. The organism maintains its integrity by processes of defense and psychological maneuvers, which in their totality are the symptoms of neurosis.

When John Spiegel and I returned from military service in 1946, some five years before our new institute was ready for occupancy, we were housed in temporary quarters where we began a fifteen-year program on stress and anxiety. Our war experiences had intrigued us, and we were concerned that they were also relevant to problems of civilian life.

For some years, we were actively concerned with a program of research designed to achieve a better understanding of anxiety in its psychological, physiological, and psychiatric expressions and to study the ways in which it develops and is handled. Central to this research was concern with "free" anxiety—the consciously experienced and subjectively reportable feelings of dread and foreboding, recognizable as internally derived and unrelated to external threats. We conceived this to be the psychological representation of a total biological state in which highly complex and interrelated changes occur at each level of organismic functioning. It was our hope that increased knowledge of this state would contribute directly to a better understanding of psychiatric disease and eventually to the improvement of treatment methods.

The investigators in this program constituted a multidisciplinary group formed with the goal of cooperating in a central program of research. With a team having diverse backgrounds in psychiatry, psychology, physiology, and biochemistry, the development over several years of mutual understanding of the diverse theoretical and methodological orientations was difficult and time consuming. Although the development of a common philosophy still remains a continuing process, the cross-fertilization already achieved in cooperative research should continue to increase the value of the group's cooperative studies, as well as their individual research.

Concern in this group had begun with the problem of anxiety from the war experiences, in which free anxiety was seen in perhaps its purest form. Subsequent studies showed that patients with chronic free anxiety have a characteristic elevation of hippuric acid excretion, which distinguishes them from normals and other psychiatric groups alike. Further studies explored this index as it changed during psychotherapy and with experimentally induced stress and mild life stress situations; for example, students at the time of examination. The research was then extended to the study of essentially normal subjects facing more severe, although temporary, stress in a life situation. A major study investigated the effects of paratrooper training on a *variety* of psychological and biochemical processes. In this, field research subjects were studied intensively before training and were then measured almost daily while facing the novel, threatening, and dangerous experiences of paratrooper training. The subjects' experience of anxiety, various aspects of psychological functioning, and different physiological indices, independently and in relation to each other, were investigated as a function of time and the training situation and in relation to individual personality structure.

Our research program originally was undertaken because Spiegel and I felt there was a need for a methodological model applicable to general problems of psychosomatic research. If such a model were fruitful in the study of a single affective state such as anxiety, it might be utilized in studies of other affects and perhaps eventually lead to the formulation of general laws. In our first research, we chose to study anxiety because of its great importance in the economy of human existence (1954 to 1957).

Anxiety has a special role in the adjustive processes of the human organism, both as an indicator of stress and as a precursor of further stress response. We believe that anxiety is a signal to the self and others portending that organismic adjustments are being made to present or expected stress in dynamically interrelated somatic, psychological, and behavioral processes. At higher levels of anxiety, as in the holocaust of war and unexpected catastrophe, equilibrium becomes so disorganized that adequate behavior, psychological efficiency, and somatic functions are profoundly disturbed. However, milder anxiety is of great significance as a *signal of threat* to the organism, for it precedes or accompanies active preparation for adjustment and, hence, may lead to facilitation of functioning at all levels.

Psychologically, the *defensive responses* may be seen in such maneuvers as counterphobic activity; magical, ritualistic behavior or thought; withdrawal; or character alteration. Thus, anxiety in some past time may be responsible for the development of psychiatric syndromes and personality deformations. Threatening recrudescence in the present, it may intensify the previous defenses or evoke new types of defenses, for free anxiety is one of the most unendurable afflictions of man. As a signal of danger, anxiety is accompanied by a host of interrelated somatic processes that are in the nature of activities preparatory to emergency action. Often, these are patterned in individual ways that derive from the subject's early learning. Whatever the later stimulus, the *personal* pattern is evoked and recognized. With decrease in psychological defenses and lessened control, anxiety mounts, and the somatic responses tend to become less discrete and patterned and more diffuse, global, and undifferentiated. Similarly, the same dedifferentiation of function can be seen in cognitive, conative, and behavioral processes as the defensive utilization of the anxiety signal breaks down.

Free anxiety can be identified as an affect in interpersonal behavior, and as such, it is objectively experienced by the subject and communicated by him to an observer. Such anxiety is experienced as an inexplicable foreboding of danger or disintegration. As an emotional experience, it is necessarily conscious and pressing. We are less concerned here with the condition termed *unconscious anxiety* or with the study of affects that are not reportable. Anxiety can best be defined by the existence of a particular emotional experience. It is relatively meaningless to speak of unconscious anxiety, intending an affect that would be present if some defense were weakened or some mode of action prohibited. Unfortunately, much psychosomatic research has been based on assumed affects that were only vaguely implicit in unconscious and underlying processes, expressed only indirectly in symbolic form.

Still, as Spiegel and I found in our paratrooper studies, the state in which anxiety is nascent or latent may be related to certain chronic states of somatic activity, and this problem requires study in its own right. What we mean to suggest is that research in this area requires a clear and consistent definition of anxiety; which should have its referent in emotional experience, rather than being an inferred psychological state from symbolic processes or from physiological concomitants.

The distinction between types of anxiety is properly made in terms of the parameters of personality discoverable in the subject. We believe it important to define different qualities of anxiety in terms of the time of onset and the life history of the individual, the ego-structure, and specific conflict areas. Such research attempting to describe various qualitative aspects of anxiety and their possible relations to qualitatively different physiological states, is necessary and important. However, for the subject himself, anxiety is phenomenally unitary, in the sense that he experiences dread and foreboding, no matter what its origin or history. Therefore, we now tentatively conceive of anxiety as being a monistic affect and attempt, through the study of personality structure, to tease out such differences existing in its qualities.

Unfortunately, the research patients with free anxiety "dried up" as the age of anxiety became the *age of defense against anxiety,* but there is some suggestion that anxiety in general is increasing as the problems of living gain in complexity. Nevertheless, in the latter part of our research program, we were forced to use emergency situations productive of anxiety such as the paratrooper experiment to provoke anxiety in some individuals in a transactional interview.

It was my experience with stress experiments that compelled me (in 1958) to become interested in a study of healthy young male adults, because I was astonished by the capacity for adequate adjustments that these subjects had exhibited, and which I predicted they would continue to exhibit if the experiences of later life were propitious. The subjects were students at George Williams College, which was operated by the YMCA. I have alluded to this experience and to this group of young adults in Chapter 7.

First, the young men were not neurotically ill or latently psychotic. Their intelligence was in the median range, with IQs of approximately 110 to 115. They revealed no evidence of having been introduced to any of the fine arts or other cultural aspects of American life. Their language was extremely simple and their vocabulary relatively meager. Their teachers had a great deal of difficulty deciphering their writing, spelling, and syntax. Conceptually, they had a great deal of trouble in dealing with abstract subjects; they were concrete people, down-to-earth, and interested in studies that have practical application. They were from upper-lower- or lower-middle-class backgrounds. They worked early in life, beginning by peddling newspapers, delivering milk, caddying on weekends, and doing miscellaneous summer jobs. This work sometimes was necessary for the economic well-being of the family, but often it was encouraged so that they would learn the value of "working for a dollar" and could earn their own spending money. Their families were characterized by their firm and consistent discipline. There was rarely any discord between the father and the mother regarding the boundaries of permitted freedom. The family itself was homogeneous, and there was very little conflict within it. Through the influence of either the father or the mother, the subject had a sound religious training in one of a wide variety of faiths. The group were Protestant, on the whole, but there were also a few Catholics and some Jews, the latter being more ambitious.

Early in life, the boys developed an interest in athletics and persisted in these activities. One of the most important characteristics of this group is their use of physical activity in coping with the disconcerting affects of anxiety or depression, or even anger. They go out onto the basketball or tennis courts and throw a few balls around or they run or swim. These are not people who sit and introspect regarding the sources of their feelings but attempt quickly to disperse them by physical activity.

The students enter George Williams College with rather firm goals and are determined to achieve them. They want to be good in their chosen field, but they have little ambition for upward mobility. They do not expect to earn more than their fathers. They have no concerns for material things; they consider their father's incomes sufficient to give them a house to live in, good clothes, good food, and possibly a second-hand car. They often stated without complaint that they had enough and did not want for anything.

Their intention to become group and activity leaders usually developed through *strong identifications* made early in life with YMCA secretaries. The YMCA has a system of hierarchical indoctrination. Gradually, the boys are screened through various activities until finally, in high school, the selected few are sent to George Williams with partial or total scholarships. The strong identification with the YMCA secretaries leads them to attempt to emulate their careers. However, such identifications are not new, as previous mechanisms indicated admiration and a firm identification with the father.

This firmly entrenched capacity for identification with one or two males has some significance for the steadfastness and stability of the group as a whole. Nevertheless, it has resulted also in constriction of interests and the tendency to report (somewhat compulsively) an action-oriented life. It is my impression that these young men are well adjusted for the particular environment in which they have fortunately been inducted. One gets the feeling that the transactional processes that lead to identification with roles suitable for a *variety* of situations are minimal. I would predict that, tempted or pushed into other environments, these boys would not look so healthy as they do at the present.

I was subsequently struck by the realization that when this group was compared with students at the University of Chicago, they were often considered deviant. When they occasionally took courses there, they were derogatorily labeled by faculty members as "upright young men." It was in an analysis of social science students at the University of Chicago, in fact, that I came across the term *the muscular Christians,* and this has always seemed to me to be an apt phrase for this group of young men with an interest in physical activity or decisive action and a missionary concept of a goal-directed life. This preliminary study started my interest in the healthy young adult, and so the next year my son and I went back to the school and tested, by means of a questionnaire devised for this purpose, 120 of the males who entered the freshman class in the fall of 1959. In addition I interviewed 40 members of this class. The correlations between questionnaires and interviews were extremely high. They revealed that the young men came from small towns in which the father was a laborer or white-collar worker. The family life was peaceable, with little discord among the parents, and the subjects felt security and love. The parents were somewhat compulsively concerned with neatness and orderliness and early toilet training. The boy was usually a favorite of the mother, but he identified with the father. There was some bickering over money, yet there was satisfaction with the father and love for him.

The boys know what to expect in the form of punishment, and boundaries are clearly defined. Discipline is consistent. The ideals of the family life are contentment, responsibility, and status quo, with little emphasis on money or fame as objects of achievement. The early hobbies are team sports in which the subjects are not usually the leaders. Aside from music, there is no interest in culture, entertainment, or in intellectual stimulation. There is a certain amount of adolescent parent-child conflict, with the parents believing that their sons should be more responsible. The youths had, however, no trouble with outside authority and show no evidence of delinquency as adolescents.

There is a *positive self-image*—the young men consider themselves, upright, honest, and responsible, with sound convictions. There had been no stormy period or emotional turmoil in their lives. Their focus and interest is on their schoolwork, and their lives are free from any crises other than preparation for examinations, which evoke only short-lived anxieties.

As the earlier study showed, these subjects seemed by background and experience to fit the norm of what is usually called healthy or normal, *as long as they remain in the environment to which they are suited.* In order to avoid the terms *healthy* and *normal,* which imply value judgments and depend on the type of transaction between personality and environment, I identified them as *homoclites,* indicating people who do not deviate from the ordinary, as do the *heteroclites.* Groups to which I presented the study saw these subjects as sick and destined to become hospitalized, for they had little ambition, cared little for money, and "wanted to do good." Absence of introspection was also deemed a cardinal sin. Further study was made in 1970, through interviews, questionnaires, and an analysis of the college records of 134 men.

An analysis of the questionnaires documents the facts that: (1) The mentally healthy young men of 1958 to 1959 have as a group sustained their good health into the third decade of their adulthood and (2) the respondents from the classes of 1960 through 1964 are similar to the respondents to the class of 1958 to 1959. In neither group were there signs of disorders in categories that give rise to mental illness. Although a few cases of mental ill health were found, the responses of the two groups can be safely considered as similar, without creating any distortion in the resulting distribution. The summation of the two sets of respondents creates a normal control with a number of the 134 men open to use by other investigators (Grinker, 1967).

In sum, *normality and illness are only polarities of a wide range of integrations;* without any strains, an unlikely hypothetical condition, there is only normality. When strained, the organismic systems respond according to the processes by which the many subvariances have become integrated. There are few new defenses or coping devices—they have already been built into the organism. Thus, the degree of health or illness in the stress responses reveals the quality and quantity of integration.

One of the characteristics of stress responses is its relation to age. Each phase of the life cycle—childhood, adolescence, young adulthood, old age and their subdivisions—has its own general predispositions, types of response, and coping devices. For example, the adolescent is concerned with moving from child– to adulthood, based on the maturation of his sex drives. The young adult is confronted with career choices. The middle-aged are concerned with discrepancies that have occurred between potentialities and accomplishments. The older subject worries about death and dying. Despite these generalities, all phases are exposed to meaningful stress stimuli in the form of anxiety, grief, loss of loved ones, feeling of hopelessness, and helplessness (giving up). All these result in somatic reactions dependent on the person's response specificity, which is innate or has been conditioned in early life.

Published studies of so-called normal personalities are extremely rare. There have been several attempts at defining so-called normality or mental health, but none of these is derived from sound empirical experience. All of them are indecisive as to who can be described as a normal personality, even within a single culture. Longitudinal studies are difficult to conduct; they are time consuming, costly, and usually last through the lifetimes of several investigators. Experience has proven that the collection of data without analysis and reporting at frequent intervals inevitably results in completely forgotten information.

Since no one is normal in an absolute sense, all of us have a degree of mental disturbance that plagues others enough to be considered sickness. In total personalities, we have character defects, minor psychopathic trends, and patterns of personality functions that appear over and over again in appropriate situations. All of us recognize the personality pattern of members of our families and neighbors, although in most cases they are not considered illnesses. Each of us is bound by a "repetition compulsion" to a recognizable life-style.

It is important to know that each of us is subjected to minor and transient episodes of anger, anxiety, and depression—even elation stimulated by episodes meaningful to us. This does not mean that we are sick and need help: We are being human—or what might be called *normally neurotic.*

In our time, interest has been revived in one aspect of mental health described by scientific investigators rather than by mental hygiene propagandists. This is the study of ways in which children and young adults cope with their human and physical environments (Murphy, 1962). From such studies, a great deal might be learned regarding health and sickness.

Do *defense* and *coping* refer to different processes or to two aspects of the same process? The basic aspect of human behavior is adaptation, which may take the form of defensive maneuvers or restructuring. The latter is called *coping* (1974, 1967). It would appear that the terms *defense* and *coping* are confounded in the psychiatric literature, inasmuch as they actually imply the same basic processes. Adaptation is the response of the biological system to stresses, but it can also in another sense refer to change in the environment. Thus, there are *allo–* and *autoplastic* adaptations, both relating to survival. The prototype of defense appears to be a response to anything impinging on the organism, whether this is from within (as an impulse) or from without. Coping seems to have the general significance of a cognitively planned, consciously contrived effort to deal with stress. The distinction between defense and coping, however, is extremely hard to maintain, for many coping attempts are not deliberately thought out, but are as compulsive as defensive behaviors. Thus, in attempts to deal with impending death, if one is prevented from using those devices that appear to be rational and deliberate, anxiety will arise, just as surely as anxiety will arise if one prevents a patient from making use of his typical modes of defense.

Perhaps coping refers to the more or less successful outcome of defensive behaviors. Hamburg and Adams (1967) originally studied applicants to the psychoanalytic institute immediately after their first selection interview. Rather than showing crippling anxiety, they actually showed a low degree of anxiety. Some applicants deliberately thought of some experiences in which they were successful. Some went around window shopping. There seemed to be a conscious, deliberate plan to cope with the anxiety. One may regard these, however, as determined by the defensive system, and what was observed was actually a successful behavioral defense against anxiety.

Hamburg and Adams (1967) outlined twenty common stressful experiences requiring adaptation: (1) separation from parents in childhood; (2) displacement by siblings; (3) childhood experiences of rejection; (4) illness and injuries in childhood; (5) illness and death of parent; (6) severe illnesses and injuries of the adult years; (7) the initial transition from home to school; (8) puberty; (9) late school transitions, e.g. from grade school to junior high school and from high school to college; (10) competitive graduate education; (11) marriage; (12) pregnancy; (13) menopause; (14) necessity for periodic moves to a new environment; (15) retirement; (16) rapid technological and social change; (17) wars and threats of wars; (18) migration; (19) acculturation; (20) social mobility.

There are suggested classes of conditions or stimuli evoking coping processes. They are subject to change as our knowledge of the human system increases. They do not include, however, the vast number of apparently simple experiences that can have significant personal meaning. Gardner Murphy (1947) sees these in more "physical" terms and identifies three classes of conditions relating to stress: (1) the need to preserve tissue, (2) strain in preparation for a stress situation, and (3) response to challenges.

To maintain a systems approach, I would tend to classify adaptation according to the components of the biopsychosocial system. All adaptation at lower levels represents phases of conflict, perturbation, or change from idling to active states. These at a higher level are invisible but appear integrated. Biologically we adapt in order to survive as individuals and as species. At the psychological level, we also cope to develop and maintain self-esteem, self-identity, and object-relations. The biological roots in primates and other infrahuman species extend by evolution to psychological methods based on new symbolic systems. At the social level, we learn how to tolerate frustrations imposed by society and to accept delay of gratification. We incorporate by identification and develop a repertoire of social roles that our culture requires.

The complexities of the meanings of the environment and the facets of the person, who must be concerned with the person-environment fit, are numerous. Demands, supplies, needs, and values all transact in the total process of adjustment.

CHAPTER 9

Depressions

THE TERM *depression* has several meanings: *moods* varying in degree and duration; a *symptom* existing behind several clinical entities (especially the psychopathies); and a *specific syndrome,* sometimes associated with mania. The effort to determine whether the syndrome is genetically and physiologically based or psychogenetic and reactive has resulted in an unfortunate dichotomy and in such false terms as *endo–* and *exogenous.* The combination of mania and depression (experienced at different times) has created the concepts of bi– and unipolar illnesses. In trying to see elements in many independent disorders that are similar, we have tried to approach depression through systems theory, and by studying cognitive, behavioral, and physiological components, as well as depressive affects.

Depression as a hereditary disease that occurred in certain families, in chronic form and often alternating with mania, occupied Kraepelin's (1910) attention for decades. Neuropathological studies were unsuccessful in locating essential lesions. Kraepelin also described some depressions that involved cognitive deterioration. Only recently has depression been linked with schizophrenia, and this linkage has affected diagnoses and has resulted in the evasive term *schizoaffective schizophrenia.* Depression has also been identified as an element in pseudoneurotic schizophrenia and in one of the phases of recovery from schizophrenic psychoses. Depression has continued to be difficult to separate from the loneliness of the borderline syndrome.

Some of the many theories and descriptions of depression can be expressed in descriptive shorthand: "the shadow of a lost loved object falls on the ego" (Mendelson, 1960); "frustration-giving ego tension" (Bibring, 1953) ; "giving up, given up (Scott and Senay, 1973) ; "assumption of responsibility for failure, separation and/or object loss (Benedek, 1956) ; "death of parent and deficient bereavement" (Beck, 1967) ; and narcissistic vulnerability and biologically deficient norepinephrine.

The psychiatric literature on depression is extensive. Abraham (1960) wrote of repressed hostility in oral characters, although currently we see many angry depressives (Lincoln was one). Bowlby (1961) contends that during the early phases of development it is not the disappointment of oral supplies that is important but the frustration of affectional needs. Attachment to the mother, he believes, is a social bond, the loss of which results in weeping, anger, and apathetic mourning in the infant. Freud (1917) wrote that loss of object-relations results in the introjected shadow of the object falling on the ego, which becomes the target of hostility (now directed inward, though originally directed toward the object).

Throughout the various theoretical formulations about depression, a number of terms are more or less universal: *repressed aggression, guilt, atonement, orality, introjection, identification,* and *self-esteem.* The subtle differences in these theoretical formulations are less significant than their adherence to the reification of concepts. Rado (1956) wrote about the despairing cry for love and narcissistic needs, which creates guilt, atonement, and forgiveness. Others considered anxiety about genitality a source of regression to the oral stage. Melanie Klein (1948) wrote about the universal depressive position of all infants, observing that those who could not introject good objects were unable to retain their self-esteem. Bibring (1953) also wrote about the loss of self-esteem that occurs when the ego is helpless to achieve success.

Jacobson (1954) considered the depressed subject to be intolerant of disappointment. Thus, the self becomes the loved object, with withdrawal from reality and loss of self-esteem, based on pathological development of the ego and superego. Aaron Beck (1967) pointed out, as have I, that proneness to defeat, devaluation of the self, and a negative view of the future constitute more than an affective process, but also include physiological and behavioral changes. Winokur (1969) has developed a theoretical etiological "spectrum": He finds in the family history of depressives alcoholism, sociopathy, blood dyscrasias, and color blindness. Identification is not always clear-cut, however, since, unfortunately, the definition of alcoholism and sociopathy is vague and varies with different ethnic groups.

It is difficult to isolate the specific factor or factors that precipitate depression, although early repetitive disappointments, sulk-prone personalities, and obsessional neurotic backgrounds clearly seem to play roles as precursors. Mendelson (1974) states that depressions are multifaceted syndromes or disorders involving cognitive, behavioral, and physiological components, as well as depressive affect. Beck's (1967) triad of psychological processes includes decrease in self-esteem and loss of confidence in the future, both of which lead to cognitive distortion.

There is some suggestion that a shift in central control is involved, in that higher-level cortical physiological functions are weakened prior to the suicide of depressed patients. Tabachnick's (1973) studies of fifteen suicides revealed that twelve had been drinking heavily before the end, contrasted with a ratio of nine of fifteen in accidental deaths. Barbiturates or other medication to promote sleep are frequently ingested chronically or in excess before the suicide. On the other hand, sleeplessness due to anxiety, with or without depression, may also be the final presuicidal precipitant. If this hypothesis is correct, the task becomes one of control of cortical vigilance without sacrificing sleep.

I do not know—despite lengthy clinical experience that included an average expectable suicide rate—what the dynamics are that pushes the patient from *thought to action,* just as I do not know the final precipitating factors for depression itself. Perhaps we would find it easier and possibly more satisfying if we discussed suicide from philosophical, existential, or moral points of view. Unfortunately, these considerations of the meaning or worth of life leave unsolved the question of the ontogenesis of hope and its accompanying illusions, which every man needs if he is to maintain value and purpose and let natural events take care of the dying.

Depressions are common among most people at some time in the wake of universal frustrations and disappointments. But these are usually mild and short-lasting. Severe depressions requiring hospitalization constitute 15 percent of state hospital admissions and 50 percent of private hospitalizations. The ratio of females to males has been 2 to 1. Hopelessness, sadness, and boredom with their roles as mothers or housekeepers appear to characterize most of the female depressions, and the cessation of goal-seeking creative ambitions and the diminishment of sexual and procreative functions characterize those of males.

On the other hand, depression may be the first sign of an undiscovered fatal illness, such as malignancy, or the first indication in a young person of an impending schizophrenic breakdown. In the elderly, removal from jobs or old neighborhoods and the death of relatives may give rise to depression as a reaction to "giving up."

Insomnia, hypochondriasis, alcoholism, and hopelessness suggest the possibility of hidden *suicidal ideas.* They can be brought out into the open by direct questioning and can be treated with adequate medication. Patients who are not willing to discuss suicidal intent are determined to kill themselves and cannot be prevented. An open expression or determination or promise not to commit suicide within a specified time gives the therapist a reasonable opportunity to treat the primary cause.

Depressions were described in ancient writings, even as far back as the first century A.D., and the descriptions differed little from those of today. In the Bible, Job's vivid portrayal of his malaise is an example. In varying degrees, patients are sad, dejected, and apprehensive. They are overwhelmed by doubts, fears, and self-accusations, some even referring to misdeeds of decades before. They also hypochondriacally, complain of numerous physical symptoms. But, they are sleepless, awakening in the morning to feel at their worst, improving at night as the day of uselessness is at an end. Appetite is diminished, and many lose much weight. Depressives express hopelessness and helplessness, and lose faith and optimism for any improvement. Some are agitated, pacing up and down asking the same questions repeatedly, as if wanting reassurance, but not listening to the answers.

There is no question that some depressions run in families and thus have a significant biogenetic (hereditary) factor. It is clear, however, that there may also be an environmental factor. Members of the family who have depressions may serve as a source of identification and become a model for the developing child. Typical of the early premorbid signs are the sulk-prone reactions of the child to early disappointments with which healthy children easily cope. However, it is increasingly recognized that overt typical depressive syndromes occur in young children.

The familial incidence of depression and mania suggest a strong *biogenetic factor* related to the cyclicity of the illness. The catecholamines (secreted by the adrenal medulla) have been implicated. It has been suggested that low concentrations of norepinephrine in the brain are related to depression and high concentrations to mania. MAO is often given to inhibit the oxygenation of norepinephrine. These hypotheses determine our choice of drug treatment. However, manic depressives also show an abnormal diabeticlike blood sugar. Thus, they are variable in mood, in glucose metabolism, and in response to psychotropic drugs. This suggests that the basic component is an *inherited hormonal variability* that requires shifts in mode of treatment during the patient's lifetime.

Currently, it is known that many neurotics are depressed and that other depressives are psychotic. Some are uni– and others bipolar (experiencing mania plus depression).

Progress toward more accurate clinical definition of the depressive syndrome (as well as of other entities) and isolation of subcategories of this global construct have been slow. It is only from developing empirically sound subcategories of depression that it is possible to make a meaningful correlation with nonpsychological data that can further knowledge of etiology, course, prognosis, and therapy.

My own interest in depression was undoubtedly related to my own recurrent mild attacks. It seems to have stemmed in large part to conversations between my father and his colleagues, which, as I recall, took place with great frequency as I was growing up. "Is your son going to be a doctor?" "Yes, he will be a neuropsychiatrist too, but *much better than I*." Over and over I heard this *better than*, until it became like a "monkey on my back" and drove me on, despite all of my handicaps and difficulties, to learn certain necessary subjects in college, premedicine, and medical school. There was nothing easy for me—my paternal superego had to be satisfied as to quantity and quality, or depression would overtake me—and it often did, but never as a syndrome preventing me from working.

My own multidisciplinary research on anxiety and stress (1955), outlined in Chapter 8, was in essence an endeavor to re-evaluate the specificity theory of Franz Alexander. Indeed, it pointed up the necessity of abandoning his *stimulus specificity* and replacing it by *response specificity.* Though it was possible to expand our affective stimulus to include anger, depression was difficult to study and measure because neither the experimental subjects nor the observers could easily determine how much depression was spontaneous and how much was stimulated by the interviewer.

When I discovered that the research group wanted to continue the original research methods without change and when federal regulations for "informed consent" threatened to negate the possibility of surprise stress, I broke up the group. In 1953, I started a new group for the study of depression, but soon realized that the psychoanalysts who were included could only discuss the dynamic theories of Freud (1913), Abraham (1960), and other analytic pioneers. Therefore, in 1954, I started a fresh group including only young psychiatrists, psychiatric residents, and a statistician, despite the fact that we had hoped to avoid the necessity of doing statistical research.

It soon became clear, however, that empirical clinical research requires numbers that cannot be simply scanned and demands the use of complicated statistical methods (Grinker, 1961).

Progress toward more accurate clinical definition of the depressive syndrome (as well as of other entities) and isolation of subcategories of this global construct have been slow. It is only from *empirically sound subdivisions of depression* that it is possible to make a meaningful correlation with nonpsychological data that can further our knowledge (Grinker, 1966b).

My phenomenological study had three major objectives: an improvement in the clinical definition of depression; the establishment of meaningful subgroups; and a determination of why patients became depressed.

There had been many shortcomings in research that had not been overcome by the previous methodology: the difficulty conceptualizing behavior patterns in the mentally ill; the elusiveness, when faced by unbiased inquiry, of definitive premorbid personality, precipitating factors, and unstereotyped psychodynamics; the pathetically inadequate routine hospital records, which in no way can be entrusted for use in clinical research, necessitating the development of new sources of information for each clinical problem; and the nonrelatedness of clinical depression with physical disease.

In a previous study of depressions, a single precipitating event was rarely isolated. Instead, a number of severe personal disappointments or stresses were observed, and the psychodynamic constellations evidenced during depressed episodes showed varied behavioral expressions.

From this, it may be observed that formulations involved during the psychoanalytic investigations of depressives are not representative of causes, except as stressors long before the onset, which are later augmented as part of the depressive process. I postulate the following circle of events: (1) Through a series of variable precipitating events, the inner conflicts and unresolved problems or unrealistic techniques of problem solving weaken a susceptible ego. (2) The ego-depletion weakens the ego's problem-solving functions, further narrows its span of control, and exposes those conflicts intensified by external problems and primarily contributing to weakening a susceptible ego. (3) The ego-depletion and regression is documented by the loss of esteem and feeling of hopelessness.

In my son's and my studies of 120 depressed patients, we have established the existence of five factors or patterns descriptive of their feelings and concerns. It is emphasized that any single patient may show evidence of more than one of these factors; they are not mutually exclusive, nor do they attempt to illustrate all aspects of any single patient.

These factors may be roughly characterized as follows: (I) a feeling of hopelessness, helplessness, failure, sadness, unworthiness, guilt, and internal suffering. There is a self-concept of "badness;" (II) a concern with material loss and an inner conviction that this feeling state (and the illness) could be changed if only the outside world would provide something; (III) guilt over wrong doing, wishes to make restitution, and a feeling that the illness was brought on by the patient himself and is deserved; (IV) "free anxiety"; and (V) envy, loneliness, martyred affliction, secondary gain with gratification from the illness, and attempts by provoking guilt to force the world into making redress.

Admitted depressed and discharged depressed patients were high in factors I and IV. Patients admitted with other diagnoses but discharged as depressed were high in factor I and low in IV. Those who were admitted with depressions but discharged with another diagnosis were low in factor I and high in IV, and those who on admission and discharge were not depressed showed only greater than average dependency on factor V. The clinical interpretation of these factors suggests that factor I is the essence of depression, and hence, its strength indicates the depth of the affective disturbance. The anxiety factor, IV, seems to indicate activity in the process and is perhaps also a signal of mobilizing or declining unconscious aggression. On the other hand, the remaining factors indicate varying attempts at defense and resolution of the depression. Hence, factor II indicates the projective defense; III, the restitution resolution; and V, the attempt by enslavery of external objects to deny anger and secondarily to regain love. The control groups seem to show that the diagnosis of the depressive syndrome is contingent not only on the depressed in the presence of minimum sadness, anxiety is enough to weigh heavily for the diagnosis of depression. Finally, the nondepressed patient whose admission diagnosis was accurate also displays dependency and demand for secondary gain.

In our series of 120 depressed patients, we have established the existence of ten factors derived from the *current behavior* checklist. These factors tend to be less sharp and distinct than the *feelings and concerns* factors, which reflect our finding that behavior is an area of less interest to psychiatrists and that our behavioral observations are not as accurate as our observations of content. Like the other factors, they are not mutually exclusive, and any single patient may exhibit a number of them. These behavioral factors may be roughly characterized as follows: (1) feelings of isolation, withdrawal, and apathy; (2) retardation, slowing of thought processes and speech; with little regard for personal appearance; (3) general retardation in behavior and gait, but less isolation and withdrawal than factor 1; (4) angry, provocative, and complaining behavior; (5) somatic complaints, including dizzy spells and constipation; (6) an "organic" concentrated, and limited and repetitive thought content; (7) agitation, tremulousness, and restlessness; (8) rigidity and psychomotor retardation; (9) somatic symptoms, such as dry skin and hair, along with some abnormalities on physical examination; and (10) ingratiating behavior, attempts to help patients and staff, and showing appreciation for the interest of the staff and the facilities of the hospital.

Correlations *between* factors derived from each checklist revealed obvious relationships but nothing striking. On the other hand, there were no correlations between the two sets of factors from the two trait lists. Again, it must be concluded that feelings are not expressed by specific behaviors: Behaviors are individually predetermined ways of responding and are not closely related to the central or basic core process of the type of depression.

Factor *patterns* were developed from the combination of fifteen factors from both trait lists. As a result, four factor patterns were elicited from which clinical profiles can be described to serve as fairly sharp hypotheses for future testing. The factor patterns are as follows:

1. *Feelings:* dismalness, hopelessness, loss of self-esteem, and slight guilt feelings
   Behavior: isolation, withdrawal, apathy, and slow speech and thinking with some cognitive disturbances
2. *Feelings:* hopelessness with low self-esteem, considerable guilt feelings, and much anxiety
   Behavior: agitation and clinging demands for attention
3. *Feelings:* abandonment and loss of love
   Behavior: agitation and demanding hypochondria
4. *Feelings:* gloom, hopelessness, and anxiety
   Behavior: demands, anger, and provocativeness

When careful psychiatric workups were done and were discussed in conference, we rarely saw a depression with a single, clear-cut precipitating event or experience. We almost invariably found a series of events that led up to the clinical illness. We also found that it was rare for the research group to reach a consensus on a formulation of the patients' psychodynamics.

Although we were unable to attribute the depression of a particular person to a specific factor or factors—i.e. premorbid personality, precipitating factors, and specific psychodynamics—we were able to subdivide the syndrome into subcategories. Included in our findings were the factors that seemed basic to depressions in general (factor I with despair and hopelessness and factor IV anxiety), and which seemed to indicate either regressive or progressive activity. The remaining factors probably indicate types of syndromes characterized by modes of defense against and resolution of the depressive affect.

That imagined object loss precedes the onset of a wide variety of physical illnesses has recently been proposed by Schmale (1958). Yet, none of our depressed patients was plagued by more than transient symptoms, such as constipation, dry mouth, or decreased serum secretion. Even the patients who were purest in the psychosomatic factor showed no evidence of somatic disease. Schmale, of course, correlates depressions with somatic illness or its onset, but the hopelessness and feelings concerning object loss are identical with traits in our source list. Does the depressive affect substitute for or protect against physical illness, or are long-term follow-up studies necessary to establish the relationship? At any rate, we were unable to confirm Schmale's findings.

Our research has developed a number of factors: five "feelings and concerns," ten "current behaviors," and, combining the two sets, four "factor patterns." These are now available for correlations with demographic data, variations in premorbid personality, type of onset, precipitating factors, physical disease and course; amenability to psychotherapy, shock therapy, pharmacotherapy, and milieu therapy; and prognosis, relapses, and accurate physiological, endocrinological, biochemical, and EEG measurements. The ultimate goal is to understand and really prevent human suffering. We may indulge those who say otherwise, with the realization that they do not understand.

Over the years, clinicians have made a host of descriptive statements based on sound observation, even better than those extant today. They have described depression, which is not a concept. It is a *disease,* and people suffer from it. The visible aspect of clinical psychiatry requires a new look at our nosological classification. We must develop rating scales and must indicate what is to be included and what is to be excluded. Eventually, all subsystems will have to *make sense clinically.* Our changing system of classification has always been difficult. It is not any cheaper than biochemical research. It is capable, at the present time, only of reliability—and that is not difficult to achieve. But validity requires relationships, the result of systems external to its own. If it does not, one or the other must be modified or discarded. Ages, sexes, and many other variables show a variety of differences. Even the use of modern hospital records is futile because of the amount of absent data. Phenomenal studies require for each research not only their own design, but their own clinical protocol. This is why the Iowa 500 is not satisfactory.

Longitudinal studies are, of course, extremely valuable, but they require a life capacity of individual observers far beyond their longevity.

Another method is the use of cross sections within sharply demarcated and described elements of the life cycle. Each phase has its own rate of growth, its own susceptibility, and its own coping devices, and each phase of the life cycle brings its own characteristics to the phenomena of depressions.

I would say that one of the most important kinds of data that could be utilized and acquired from study of the phases of the age cycle are biological differences that exist when individuals are *not* depressed. One can conclude that they are independent of the mood, the affect, and the disease. Some of the material on the lack of delta sleep, regardless of the presence of depression, seems to be important in that respect.

The depressive mood is characteristic of many psychological states, not only of the syndrome of depression. The latter includes rhythmic appearances and manic attacks, etc. As is true of all excited phases, including catatonic excitement, the so-called psychotic depressions are definitely decreasing in frequency, at least in the United States, as contrasted to the United Kingdom. Instead, restricted-constricted characters have increased all over the world. Depression as a mood is one of the few characteristics, however, of human responses under stress situations.

The problems of change in systems of communication, not as one of the causes but probably as a result, bring up the question of the concomitants or indices. Whatever the cause, the effect of disturbances in communication on the various indices, such as dry mouth, constipation, and so on, are time limited on an individual basis, except, and this is important for the study of people of older ages, when senility or arteriosclerosis catches up. Despite the duration of a given episode, from the depression itself, there seems to be no physical residue. *During* the depression, loss of weight and hypotension occur, which contradicts Schmale's notion that "giving up" is a precursor of serious physical disease. When depression begins from whatever causes (and it is difficult, I would say almost impossible, to determine the psychological precipitating cause), it runs to its own limits.

Now there seems to be a reciprocal relationship between biochemical (pharmacological) and psychological factors. Starting at either arc of the cycle, any transaction may initiate the whole process. It can start with a biochemical or a psychological alteration, and the process can be the same, no matter where its beginning. The difficulty is in separating the indices from the more basic elements of the process (up to now we feel that they must be studied simultaneously). The levels of complexity are equal on both sides. Exact biochemical and rough clinical estimates are really not correlatable. The biochemist has the responsibility for using the clinical phenomenon, as we now know it.

In summary, it is evident that, though much work remains to be done, the direction of research into depression has become clearer. Wolpert (1977), working in our institute, has published a study on depressive illness in which he states that he considers it to be an "actual neurosis." The basic problem, he believes, is a periodic increase or lack of norepinephrine, which causes a shift in the affective system and is neutralized by lithium carbonate, not by psychotherapy alone. Conversely, only some abnormalities are triggered by psychological stimuli and can be helped by psychotherapy alone.

In a 352-page review of depressions, Mendelson (1974) surveys all the existing theories relating to this disease. He concludes, "I believe that the psychoanalytic task of understanding depression has been largely completed—But it seems to me that the significant focus of new work on depression will continue to shift in a neurophysiological and psychopharmacological direction."

CHAPTER 10

Schizophrenia

SCHIZOPHRENIA has a worldwide occurrence, although different words are used to describe its symptoms, and it is attributed to a variety of causes, from incursions by malignant agents to evil thoughts and behavior. Today, North Americans seem to be afflicted by acute schizophrenia more than in the past, but on the whole, its course, after adequate treatment, is much more benign than was reported in the last century. Many are successfully returned to the community from hospitals and many are never hospitalized, so that the rate and incidence of the disease cannot be accurately determined.

One of the best-known of the so-called radical psychiatrists, Thomas Szasz, seems to call into doubt the existence of schizophrenia. His multiple papers and books repeat what seems to be a profitable tune. I quote from his latest work, *Schizophrenia: The Sacred Symbol of Psychiatry* (1977): "Real medicine thus helps real physicians to treat or cure real patients; fake medicine (psychiatry) helps fake physicians (psychiatrists) to influence or control fake patients (the mentally sick)."

It is easy enough to dismiss Szasz. What is important is to define the phenomenology of schizophrenia so that all disciplines have an adequate referent on which to base their investigations. This is a difficult task, despite the thousands of papers and books written on the subject. In our own attempt to understand schizophrenia, we must continually reevaluate previous studies and continue further investigation with energy and dedication.

The term *psychosis* has been used in a variety of ways. One of the worst offenses is to consider psychosis and schizophrenia as synonymous. Most schizophrenics, in fact, are not psychotic, at least during long periods of their illness. In truth, psychosis is a behavioral term designating an attempt to remodel disorganized reality by means of delusions and hallucinations. Thus, psychoses are characterized by unrealistic behavior that disrupts most, if not all, forms of adaptation and seriously disorganizes personality.

In young schizophrenics experiencing their first breakdowns, the acute psychotic experience is short-lived. They seem more depressed than excited, with anhedonia and loneliness, but there is less cognitive disturbance and associative slippage. It is not known which of the significant system factors contribute most to the psychoses, i.e. biogenetic, childrearing, early physical disease, traumatic experiences, family patterns and systems of communication, life stresses, socioeconomics, or culture. Etiological articulation of biological, psychological sociological, and cultural systems is not yet possible.

Thought disorder, according to Koh (1976-1978), is a part of basic organizing processes, among which are a number of other parts that transact among each other, so that deficiencies in one part or of organizing defects cannot be considered as single courses. Furthermore, we cannot as yet specify that any weakness or defect is biologically or experientially determined or both. Aside from thought disorders, other parts include the perceptive functions that screen input or recognize feedback; the memory banks that verify the significance of thinking in terms of past experiences; feelings that modify effectiveness of thinking or are influenced by confused thoughts; and action or behaviors that express how informational input has been internally processed and organized. These parts constitute the schizophrenic system of perceptions, thoughts, feelings, and organization. Beyond the system, sociocultural factors contribute to the clarity of the input or of the appropriations or congruence of output behaviors within the social context, thereby constituting the challanges or precipitating factors involved in disorder or psychosis.

A study of the literature concerned with schizophrenia reveals repetitive statements of theory and of empirical observations of obscure relevance, producing many "little answers" that are difficult to integrate. The student soon arrives at a point or redundancy of information or "noise." The levels of complexity are so many that theories emphasizing simplicity and parsimony are too limited and those emphasizing generalities are too global. What we call *theories* are collections of related propositions, not *"facts."* Unfortunately as yet, "facts" or empirical observations on schizophrenia lack adequate precision and definition.

The problems associated with schizophrenia demonstrate clearly that there is no single cause and that multiple factors enter into every aspect of cause, course, and outcome. As a result, many theories have been constructed appropriate to various specific foci of observation or levels of interest. These necessitate different techniques of study, for which expertise in various scientific disciplines is required. Each requires concentration, technology, and language specific for its purposes. Yet, each is dependent on others, especially on clinical or empirical investigations to define *what* is being studied. The geneticist, biochemist, or physiologist, requires firm and accurate diagnoses to be sure he is studying processes of schizophrenics, their subcategories, and the state or phase of the ever-changing disturbance.

What are these many scientists studying? What is schizophrenia? These are *first* questions still not answered. For example, the combined experiences and study of the literature by several psychologists and psychiatrists forced us into an artificial consensus to develop a Michael Reese definition of schizophrenia as a temporary working hypothesis. What is needed now is a well-conceived program of study in continuity to define clinical schizophrenia and its categories that can be useful for *all* scientific studies. Briefly stated, I believe that this requires a study of verbal and gross behaviors in relatively free fields where opportunities are present for many kinds of relations with a variety of people. The focus, then, would be on what challenges, well defined, excite or ameliorate equally well-defined categories of responses? What psychological tests represent these challenges in brief or miniature encounters?

When we know more about what schizophrenia and/or its categories are, then geneticists, physiologists, chemists, psychologists and sociologists will be studying the same process. Certainly all systems, but some more than others (genetics), require behavioral referents for their correlations. Yet, today, we know that simple correlations artificially disregard defferent units of measurement and different temporal dimensions. Modern multivariate analyses require clinical phenomena and classification as the scientific backbone on which the flesh of a host of other variables may be properly positioned.

We have become increasingly aware that correlations between brain structure-function and behavior; between emotional affective responses and internal feelings and concerns; between deficient logical structures and capacities for abstract thinking; and between limited emotional and cognitive means and adaptation to reality are indeed not simple. As a result, more interest in bridging theories and models has developed.

It is not that we should discard theories appropriate to various levels of organization and experience, nor abolish specific methods of investigation. To put each in an appropriate position within a total field, so that the transactions among its parts may be defined in process terms by observations from specific frames of reference permits a larger, more correct view of any biopsychosocial system. At the same time, it does not sacrifice the hard sciences of experimentation nor the softer sciences of behavioral observations.

Are the schizophrenic response patterns specific, or are they exaggerations of common human responses to stress, as in war neuroses or in anxiety states or in other regressive, dedifferentiating processes?

Shakow (1971) points out the poor generalized preparation for input (lack of curiosity and search for stimulation) ; the poor preparation for specific input (extreme sensitivity for irrelevancies); the disturbance of actual input (unrealistic perceptions); the defect in central control involving thinking, affect, and variability, etc.; and the inadequacy of the output stage giving rise to deficient and disorganized performances. Is this the primary gestalt that differentiates the schizophrenic from the healthy? Can we unify our theoretical concepts into a single comprehensive theory that encompasses all levels of disturbed behavior?

Young first-break schizophrenics are able to maintain a good organization during unstructured and structured taped interviews, despite periods of psychotic and highly variable behavior in the nursing unit. They recount honestly and fairly completely the events of their lives, the events leading up to their breaks, and their experiences during psychotic periods with an earnest desire to help the research project into which they have entered voluntarily.

Our definition of five categories of schizophrenia are, of course, tentative, only confirmable by our planned twenty-year follow-up studies. *Acute schizophrenics* are those with sharp, rather suddenly appearing psychotic episodes who quickly enter into a remission, but often with subsequent disorganization, and who can be returned to school or jobs, their families, and social groups. *Chronic schizophrenics* usually indicate childhood experiences of inner turmoil and social incompetence, gradually developing a psychotic break. *Paranoid schizophrenics* reveal more than the general schizophrenic feeling that the world and its people are insufferable to them, but feel specifically that persons are plotting against, spying and planning evil deeds directed against them. Schizophrenics with convulsions are those with generalized fits preceding the psychotic episode. They do not have jacksonian focal epilepsy, uncinate fits, or violent ictal rage attacks. *Schizo affective disordered people* include in their life histories or during their attacks either depressions (deeper than anhedonia) or manic behaviors or both the schizophrenic thought disorders. The *nonschizophrenic* controls are patients sufficiently ill that hospitalization is warranted. So-called *normal controls* are people previously described as homoclites, as well as age-matched staff members.

Family studies reveal frequent pathology in the families of the index subjects and a frail, sad voice of the acutely ill schizophrenic and the expression and a history of chronic anhedonia, often to the depth of depression and suicidal thoughts or attempts; the high degree of dependency on the mother or her substitute ambivalently associated, with rage toward her usually unexpressed; the paucity of affectionate relations to anyone; and the recognition that the psychosis was precipitated by unattainable goals and the willingness to settle for less in life. Frequently, the first break occurred on entering college and having to compete with other highly intelligent highschool graduates.

Although the psychotic episodes were associated with severe

thought disorders (slippage, neologisms, confusion, and flooding disorder in logic) these were not permanent and seemed to become damped down thereafter, until another break occurred.

Anxiety in the presence of other people forced the subjects to remain isolated in their rooms playing a guitar, listening to their stereos, or daydreaning. Attempts at resocialization on the nursing unit gradually became more and more successful. These developed a push toward and a pull back from people until an equilibrium was reached.

When anxiety was the dominant feeling, it was associated with a foreboding of "going to pieces" or "going crazy." However, loneliness, sadness, and depression were the most frequent reported feeling states.

When the schizophrenic break is described as a period of disintegration and disorganization, it is also referred to as the weakening of a supraordinate controlling or regulatory process. Improvement is evidenced by better control or some degree of reorganization. As the patients state, "I feel that I have better control, but the difficulties I experienced are still there, but in lesser degree."

Holzman and I (1974) contend that the conflict theory applicable to the neuroses is not applicable to schizophrenia. We have compiled observational data since 1970 and do not find evidence that neuroses and psychoses represent phases of the same process. In fact, schizophrenic psychoses show a host of behavioral symptoms not seen in the neuroses. They are not to be conceived of as part of a continuum, and they cannot be studied by psychological methods alone. Kayton's (1977) analysis of the phases of recovery also clearly places the schizophrenias in a separate category from the neuroses.

Manfred Bleuler (1974), in a paper on the long-term course of the schizophrenic psychoses, states:

> Many recovered schizophrenics continued to do well even without medication and social care. As a rule, schizophrenics had no endocrine pathology and endocrine patients were not schizophrenic. Neither a broken home in childhood nor an upbringing by a schizophrenic parent resulted in any important association with schizophrenia. However, a disturbed relationship with relatives and a loved

> person was more frequent in the anamnesis of schizophrenic women than of schizophrenic men. Most schizophrenics who had been schizoid before their psychosis had lived in miserable family situations.

In our own long-term study (blind) of hospitalized young patients, we found "spin-offs" of young depressives, schizoaffectives, anorexias, paranoids, and borderlines, all of whom will be followed, just as the schizophrenics, with the same rating scales and a statistical analyses.

To indicate the background of research in schizophrenia, it is necessary only to refer to the huge compilations of the literature and the recent summarizing volumes. These indicate that a wide range of investigations have extended from biogenetic factors to sociocultural ones—yet there is little consensus. The variability that is characteristic of both individuals and groups has been discouraging; it has been used as an excuse for failure when, in fact, it constitutes an important aspect of schizophrenia itself. Aside from Bleuler's early definition, schizophrenia has been seen as potpourri of several conditions and processes, none of which has been clearly defined. As a result, correlations among variables studied by investigators from many disciplines has become exceedingly difficult, because it is never certain that it is the same phenomenon that is being studied. Thus, a primary question must be: What is the phenomenology of different types of schizophrenia?

The second question concerns the psychological—thinking, feeling, and behavioral—manifestations that may furnish clues to the underlying biological defects present in the schizophrenic. For example, is the quality of schizophrenic anxiety and thinking derived from a dysfunction of the endocrine or central nervous system, or is it a result of metabolic functions or organizational processes necessary to maintain the systems in the face of stress? The teleological meaning of the disease as an adaptation is a question usually shunned by scientists, but according to Brueke (quoted by Cannon, 1945), "Teleology is a lady without whom no biologist can live. Yet he is ashamed to show himself with her in public." We are less interested, in this research, in the personal psychodynamics (which varies from subject to subject) than in the patterning of psychological functions.

The third question that must concern us is the way in which other systems are involved or correlated with the psychological.

The fourth question concerns the variability at different times and under different conditions within individuals and groups of subjects.

MacFie Campbell (1935) stated, "I prefer to think of them [schizophrenics] as belonging to a Greek letter society, the conditions for admission to which are obscure; inclusion and exclusion from the fraternity are determined by considerations which may vary from year to year and from place to place, and the directing board is not known."

Can we ask the question "Where is *the* weakness in schizophrenia leading to disturbances in feeling, thinking, and behavior?" Not exactly: It is in fact not accurate to state the question in that form, since schizophrenia is itself a system not produced either by a polygenetic defect or by society alone. As a system, many factors are responsible at least for the preparation of the overt disease. Perhaps a weighted scale may be developed for a *continuum:* The greater the biogenetic factor, the less severe the stimulus necessary for an overt syndrome; the lesser the biogenetic factor, the stronger the stress stimulus must be. Unfortunately, a single biogenetic factor has not yet been discovered in gene studies; it has been only indirectly assumed through studies of monozygotic twins, familial incidence, biochemical alterations, and some preliminary studies of dysfunctional biological markers, such as those Holzman has discovered in eye-tracking deficits.

We can say that in a pleasureless life, in what has been called *anhedonia,* there is difficulty in maintaining organizational coherence, and there is excessive dependency and deficiency in competency well below the subject's assets in work, school, or social interactions. These deficits are accompanied by a vulnerable sense of self-regard and self-esteem, which becomes clear during and after a psychotic break. It is only in those patients who seem to be destined for a chronic course that we may uncover unmistakeable signs of psychotic behavior in early childhood.

Corresponding to the above deficiencies, the stress stimuli provoke a psychosis after a breakup in a close relationship, a loss of dependency, such as leaving home for college, or a rejection by someone important. The responses to these stress stimuli can no longer be considered as necessarily falling into the classical categories of Kraepelin (1912, 1919) and E. Bleuler (1950), etc.

Our own studies reflect a more basic, hypothetical dysfunction in maintaining the kind of organization necessary for appropriate, adaptive orientation to one's surroundings and to oneself. This basic disorder, we would further hypothesize, need not lead inevitably to psychosis. The loose adherence to stable organizations may sometimes lead to reorganizations of reality that may even have social, artistic, or scientific value. We would suppose, however, that a significant degree of competence among other factors would be necessary for such an outcome. At any rate, the acute schizophrenic may remit from his psychoses entirely or almost completely. Whether the schizophrenic thought disorder persists during this remission is still a vexing controversial problem.

We are also by no means sure that we can predict the outcome: There may be steady deteriorations, deterioration in shifts following each of several acute attacks, or repeated acute attacks with little general dedifferentiation. The end results cannot yet be predicated during the acute phase.

If schizophrenics are viewed dynamically and we become intrigued with the content of their thinking, we will end up in a blind alley of nonunderstanding. Such interpretations will harm rather than help these patients. Using Hughlings Jackson's paradigm, the loss of control and defective organization results in negative symptoms, involving relations with other systems in reality. The positive symptoms are related to the dedifferentiation or devolution, which permits previously inhibited infantile patterns to reappear.

If the clinical syndrome is an adaptive defense against the still unknown schizophrenic process, then the shutting off from reality represents an excessive defense reaction (with some lacunae) within the dereistic shell. The hallucinations and delusions then represent a substitute form of thinking more pleasurable than the reality that cannot be mastered.

A systems approach is bound to abrogate such false dichotomies or polarizations as the linear cause-and-effect concepts and the nature-versus-nurture conflicts. The position of the physician-observer or the investigator can be clearly defined in space and time, and by weighing the factors in multiple causations, he can improve his ability to focus accurately on his therapeutic goals. The student will have to accept a degree of indeterminancy and probability amidst a larger collective order.

This means that in the multivariant dynamics, change in a part of the total process of any disease is linked to its causes. Thus, parts can only be specified by their quantitative ranges. In all of medicine the question, as Paul Weiss, (1962-63) states, is not what man should do, but what he should not do to repeat his mistakes. There must be what Weiss calls a "sanitation of traditional frames of reference."

In general, theories of psychopathology have been zealously defended and have been considered to be contradictory to each other. Millon (1973) has clearly stated that theories of psychopathology should be considered as complementary, differing according to their areas of focus. He enumerates them as biophysical, intrapsychic, behavioral, and phenomenological, all specifying hypotheses concerning etiology, pathology, and treatment. Classification of theories is, however, still a matter of personal choice. Each is associated with specific levels of organization, and each contains a certain amount of dogma. As Millon states, theories should be evaluated on the grounds of simplicity and parsimony, generality of application, empirical precision, and derivable consequences. Nevertheless, a pure psychogenetic theory is as untenable as a pure genetic theory.

The numerous theoretical approaches to the problem of schizophrenia are vigorously adhered to by their special proponents. Through their hypothesis, research designs, and in general, their paradigms, seem quite different, they can be subsumed under several categories.

All the theories have not been developed a priori, but some are based on observational phenomena of which cognitive and emotional disturbances of function are apparently central. Bleuler's outstanding contribution has been the separation of primary invariant disturbances from secondary symptoms. On the basis of empirical evidence, psychoanalysts have further refined the distinction between basic anxiety and defensive and restitutive processes. Shakow (1971) has outlined his thinking concerning psychopathological theory in general. First, the phenomena are defined from objective empirical studies from which inferences and categorization can be made and theory constructed. Second, there is an attempt to develop a theory of etiology. Unfortunately, these attempts are clouded by shifting overemphasis on either meaning or on rigorous measurements devoid of meaning.

Don Jackson (1960) has attempted to categorize current theories as follows: (1) organic, (2) biological vulnerability, (3) predisposition, plus stress, (4) psychosomatic, (5) early trauma revivified, (6) maladaption of the family group, and (7) purely psychogenetic. There are several other similar summaries. I would like to propose another scheme of general theories, each one of which interdigitates with the others.

1. The *organic theories* postulate disturbances of structure-function of the central nervous system. These may be inherited or acquired and act directly on the nervous system or indirectly through abnormalities of the endocrine system (adrenals and thyroid, etc.) or through disordered metabolism.

2. The *psychological theories* are concerned with functional disturbances of mentation and feelings as end process of ontogenetic experiences.

3. *The social theories* are concerned with the direct influences of the human environment, including the family, at various levels on the learning processes during maturation.

Such overlapping of multiple factors places the theory of schizophrenia in the currently acknowledged broad *biopsychosocial* field. Among the terms used to incorporate all the approaches are *psychosomatic, multifactorial, field* and *general systems theory.* These are much more sophisticated than the usual, oversimplified two-system correlations or the hope-inspiring concept of difficulty in central control, or deficiencies in organizational processes, or the pessimistic statement that schizophrenia is an attempt to adapt to a problem that is insoluble.

Bleuler's theory was based on the proposition of primary psychological symptoms. Since then, considerable evidence has accumulated to indicate that there are somatic symptoms as well, and certainly there are multiple behavioral deviations. Since we cannot fracture the symptomatic field, the theoretical approach also requires a generalized field theory. The question is, therefore, how do we deal with the extended field conceptually and operationally?

I should like now to restate the theoretical concepts applicable to schizophrenia, breaking the *biopsychosocial* unity into its parts in an attempt at achieving a schematic chronological order.

I. *Altered Biogenic or Hereditary Background*

Some genic deviations, probably recessive, predispose the individual to adaptive difficulties because of disordered structure-function of the central nervous system or disorders of the endocrine or metabolic systems indirectly affecting the central nervous system. These do not, however, make a schizophrenic.

II. *Developmental Experiences*

Early inputs by virtue of satisfactions versus dissatisfactions, trauma versus safety, security versus threats of annihilation, and information of various quantities and consistency furnished by the mother and/or family and other members of the human environment prepare the individual for living in a stressful world and create a life-style of varying degrees of stability. These experiences acting on a prepared soil (heredity) within critical periods are more or less disturbing.

III. *Anxiety*

Inherent in the product of the interaction of the above factors are universal anxieties producing varying types of defenses, depending on the degree and timing of inputs and the quality and quantity of the anxiety. These are significant foundations on which later cues, derived from internal or external stimuli, act on the prone organism and evoke coping, integrative, or disintegrative behaviors.

IV. *Challenges*

Challenges constitute the meaningful precipitating factors acting on a prepared organism. They may be overwhelming or mild, overt or covert, or consistent or inconsistent. Yet, they expose the characteristic psychological set of the schizophrenics' neophobia, perseverations, or weakening of central control. In lesser degrees, these interactions may be exposed only by psychological test situations.

V. *Primary Symptoms*

These include disturbances of psychological associations, disturbances in affect, ambivalence, loosening of ties with reality, and recourse to fantasy life. Permutations of these and their individualized expressions have been used in the current system of classification of types of symptoms.

VI. *Secondary Symptoms*

Secondary symptoms include coping devices or defenses, compensations, and hallucinatory and delusional attempts at restitution of stability, as well as reactions to primary symptoms and to anxiety. Among the latter are aggressive attacks on the disturbing people who attempt to permeate defenses, in spite of a terrifying loneliness after withdrawal.

Any chronological ordering of these processes is artificial, because all elements are active at all subsequent times after their initial appearance. They are usually reinforced, and positive feedback mechanisms accentuate prior elements. The cycle generates intensification of the disorder, since there is no evidence of control or negative feedback mechanisms. Correspondingly, schizophrenia is not cured. It may spontaneously come to a halt, or it may spontaneously or through various interventions, be in some way alleviated. Thus, psychotherapy may accomplish a more realistic evaluation of challenges or a detachment of voluntary movement away from known stimuli to which the individual is vulnerable. Drugs may decrease central excitability, or behavioral therapy may ameliorate responses to anxiety. Some psychotherapy may open outlets for unsatisfied childish needs, and family therapy may decrease the demands on voluntary behavior. At any rate, as theories in general postulate the factors responsible for any disease—the host, the provocative agents, and the environment—so therapy may act on any one of this triad. Because the process is established before critical periods, rarely do any therapies "cure."

Because the process begins so early (denying the validity of a purely "reactive" schizophrenia) and is based on primary biological foundations that, even though latent, are probably always part of various transactions during the developmental phases and even later, field concepts require specific chronological ordering of the included parts. The systems within the schizophrenic field are not equipotential, and there is a progressive movement of parts, each one being dependent on its precursor, toward ultimate regression.

One of the mysteries embodies the universality of the primary symptom complex (thought disturbance) and the common subcategories of secondary symptoms giving rise to the existing classifications Kraepelin's or S. Beck's (1965) six schizophrenias. Are these phenomena related to the degree of anxiety? Great anxiety has a cognitive effect, as does intense depression. Conversely, is the source (quality) of anxiety the reason for the cognitive disturbance, i.e. the unmanageable world as perceived during developmental periods? Is anxiety unmanageable because of genetic factors, because it is actually too stressful, or because the object relations and ego boundaries are constitutionally so weak that the cruel world has to be internalized? Reinforcement of these processes results in the need for only minimal cues to set off the process (from time to time), thus accounting for such variability.

There is sufficient consistency in classical schizophrenia to warrant the establishment of a syndrome with subtypes. It must be admitted that the boundaries of each are weak and imperfect for any degree of reliability. Yet, we need to ask whether any of the schizophrenic phenomena are specific and unique in themselves. Cognitive disturbances, regressions, withdrawals, and anxieties are also present in neuroses, in depressions, and to some degree in the so-called healthy. If the flow of events does not include genic or constitutional factors, then regression is seen a natural psychological phenomena that anyone can utilize under certain circumstances beyond endurance thresholds. The splitting of the ego occurs even in healthy normal development. It is true that the ego is primarily split and in development is synthesized into a specific self-system and a type of life-style. Everyone needs to withdraw into isolation from time to time. Depressions and stress reactions are also associated with cognitive disturbances.

Each set of theories, and I have certainly now illustrated only their prototypes, and each combination of theories evokes specific hypotheses and questions. More important than specific questions is the need now to bring the multiple theories into an understandable fruitful synthesis. It is imperative to alleviate the competitive spirit interfering with significant multidisciplinary research. To view the theories, stated precisely in complementary form, may enable good multidisciplinary research to develop.

It was not until 1952 that childhood schizophrenia was accepted as a clinical entity, with the first paper by Loretta Bender and A.M. Freedman and the later confirmatory studies by Bender (1971). She showed that those schizophrenic children had profound disturbances in the function of their vestibular systems. They did not respond adequately to twirling and had a peculiar tonelessness in their somatic musculature.

Does schizophrenia begin in early childhood? Most of the evidence is retrospective, through interviews complicated by falsification, forgetting, and repression. Prospective longitudinal studies on high-risk children would seem to be more appropriate. On the other hand, Anthony (1969) has astutely described micro-psychotic episodes in children who later became schizophrenic.

There is extensive literature on high-risk children, monozygotic twins, and children adopted from Denmark, where controlled and identifiable populations are available. In our material, there are only a few identical and fraternal twins. Family studies attempt to ascertain the onset of peculiar behavior and family occurrence. We hope in the future to include a childhood population at a nearby children's hospital (Pritzker Children's Center).

Although a genetic component is a necessary condition, environmental pressures are necessary to make it manifest. Indeed, it may be that the genetic component or contribution to schizophrenia is no greater than the genetic contribution to the development of a neurosis or a character disorder. Finding the genetic underpinning of schizophrenia would uncover only one of the necessary conditions for the development of psychosis.

In accordance with our attempt to study schizophrenia at several phases of the disorder, one aspect of our overall project has been our research on *schizophrenia in adolescence.* We began by making a clear distinction between schizophrenia and schizophrenic psychosis.

Adolescence imposes severe demands for social and inter– and intrapersonal competence on the biological and psychologically vulnerable youngster, often causing him to retreat in some type of psychopathology.

Adolescence begins at puberty but ends at various ages. It is a biological phase of development with hormonal, sexual, and physical changes (Grinker and Holzman, 1974). It is also a culturally defined stage in the life cycle, varying with the society in which the adolescent develops and lives. In his changing roles, he searches for what he cares to do and who he cares to be. Psychologically, he may grow continuously, in spurts, or in turmoil. Therefore, several types of adaptation are required to achieve social, interpersonal, motor, and intellectual competence.

Adolescence, with its insistent demands for separation and individuation, for taking a role in society, and for performing it with competence, imposes inescapable burdens on a vulnerable organism (Grinker and Holzman, 1974). In the vulnerable person, response is weak, inappropriate, inadequate, avoidant, defiant, absent, apathetic, ineffective, desperate, eccentric, or compliant-at-great-cost.

From this perspective, it is understandable that the statistics regarding first hospitalizations for schizophrenic patients show that young males outnumber young females until the fourth decade of life, when females are in the majority. The task demands on young adult males are greater than those on young females, including requirements for competence in the social, occupational, and sexual realms. The young male must, in most cultures, establish himself in an occupation and become sexually aggressive enough to court and marry a woman, and to maintain sexual, social, and occupational potency. Thus, in men, limitations in competence become apparent early and task demands impose heavy challenges. For young women, in our culture, on the other hand, the requirements for independence and initiative are less than they are for young men. Thus, the appearance of overt disorganization—the psychotic phase of the disorder—is less apparent in young women.

In our view, then, the relationship between adolescence and schizophrenia is that of a *catalyst to a biological reaction.* The potential for disorganization is a characteristic of the person. The social tasks of adolescence, however, place powerful strains on a vulnerable youth, and such a person must draw on his finite resources to respond to these task requirements. His responses thus expose his vulnerabilities, and the strain of the requirement to become competent can potentiate disorganization. The consequences of such failures to the adolescent's sense of worth, self-esteem, and pride are great; they add finite burdens to his failures already sensed throughout the preceding years.

The common types of schizophrenia are classified by our research group into five subcategories, although there are several other classifications usable as well.

1. *Acute Schizophrenic Psychosis* characterizes people with sharp, rather suddenly and recently appearing psychotic episodes after a period of previous good adjustment, who soon enter into a remission with only a little evidence of subsequent disorganization, and who can be returned to school or jobs, their families, and their social groups.

2. *Chronic Schizophrenic Psychosis* indicates long-standing experiences of inner turmoil and social incompetence with clear psychotic symptoms, but without the necessary appearance of an acute psychosis. A gradually developing psychosis is the typical picture.

3. *Paranoid Schizophrenic Psychosis* designates those who experience frank delusions with a persecutory or grandiose content. They are not typically bizarre in their conventional behavior or even generally in their thinking, except when the focus is on delusional content. They also tend to be cautious, suspicious, and hyperalert.

4. *Schizophrenic Psychosis with Convulsions* designates those with generalized seizures preceding an acute schizophrenic psychotic episode. They do not have jacksonian focal epilepsy, uncinate fits, or violent ictal rage attacks.

5. *Schizoaffective Psychosis* describes a group who, in their life histories or during their psychotic attacks, manifest either depressions (as distinguished from anhedonia), or manic behaviors, or both, as well as schizophrenic thought disorders. These are quite difficult to diagnose (Grinker and Holzman, 1974).

Many schizophrenics are able to manage well in their usual activities and may need occasional ambulatory professional help. Others may have various degrees of disorganization, the worst of which is an acute psychosis requiring hospitalization; for them, a milieu in which they are treated with dignity and understanding and antischizophrenic drugs, such as the phenothiazines, are indicated. Psycho– group, and family therapy may be helpful. Planning for better living and lowered career goals should be made before discharge. At best, the psychosis may be terminated, but the schizophrenic tendency remains. Lobotomy and electroshock treatments are used rarely. Massive doses of vitamins are often used, but their value has not been proved.

That biological factor in schizophrenia is clearly important is evidenced by twin and family studies. There are some patients with soft neurological signs, biochemical disorders, and bioelectric abnormalities in the brain. Disorders of communication in families of schizophrenics are also frequent. Yet, both hereditary and environmental factors together are necessary to produce a schizophrenic. This should not impose pessimism in the parents. Psychiatrists now have the tools to help the schizophrenic as never before.

Although our research program at P & PI is oriented toward answering questions of definition, etiology, and adaptation, we are dealing with sick people who need treatment. The role of antischizophrenic drugs, such as the phenothiazines, is of course, a crucial question. Can they be used effectively for all kinds of schizophrenia? There is some growing evidence, for example, that the phenothiazines are not particularly effective with non-paranoid schizophrenic patients with a good premorbid history and that there may be some therapeutic advantage in not administering phenothiazine medication to these patients at some phases of the illness. But does it make clinical sense to withdraw such medication uniformly from all patients in our care?

The acute outbreak of the schizophrenic psychosis, as opposed to those cases with an insidious onset or those with a chronic course, has a particularly devastating effect on a family. What help can and should be given to them during the phase of the patient's disorganization? Can the family be treated as a group with a focus on support, understanding, and guidance, thereby perhaps preventing the outbreak of a psychotic response in yet another family member? These are questions that require further study.

A close study of a number of successfully treated schizophrenic patients permits the therapist to divide the clinical course during treatment into four phases, which have been well described by Kayton (1973), who worked with those psychotic schizophrenics on our nursing unit. Kayton describes Phase I as that of *internal disorganization,* the psychotic period.

During this period, the patient is preoccupied with sinister, powerful, persecutory forces (with bad objects and with powerful, grandiose forces). Thought slippage, flooding, and clogging are common at this phase. The patients are also preoccupied with good objects and with hopes of rescue, yet extreme vulnerability to rebuffs and feelings of panic are common. During Phase II, the phase Kayton labels *postpsychotic regression,* which occurs after the resolution of the psychosis, there are feelings of aloneness, weakness, badness, and emptiness, with many hypochondriacal concerns (and severely impaired concentration, attention, and reasoning). Withdrawal from other people is typical, as are silences during therapy sessions. Reversals of the sleep-waking pattern are typical, and shifts in body image may persist. During Phase III, *concentration begins to improve* (and disorganization begins to subside). The patients begin to become concerned about their appearances, and social relationships (begin) spontaneously (to) reappear. During this phase, regression can be terminated rather expeditiously by interpretation, firmness, and structure setting. Phase IV, that of the *termination of the regression,* is ushered in by feelings of inner strength and by the initiation of activity. A normalized diurnal cycle appears, and there is a return of some self-confidence, although it is accompanied by lowered ambitions.

It has seemed to us that during the phase of psychosis and postpsychotic regression, working with internal conflict is less appropriate than it would be during the recovery phases. (A unitary theory of neurosis and schizophrenia dictates a standard psychoanalytic technique.) Our experience shows that a classical psychoanalytic approach at the psychotic and postpsychotic phase deepens the regression and prolongs the appearance of recovery. During the early phase of the psychotic regression, techniques of making contact with and reassuring the frightened patient and of assuring proper nutrition and other health standards should receive priority. It is a real question in our minds whether the acutely psychotic schizophrenic patient "requires" a prolonged period of regression in order to recover and to heal. (We have, of course, argued within our own group about whether premature resolution of acute confusional periods may interfere with later phases of the treatment and whether there may be advantages to the patient in learning to live with his confusions for a while. We have, however, not come to any conclusion about this position. Our treatment program tries to limit the regression as best we can. This is one area where sensitive observation can contribute to a theory of psychosis in functional terms. (We allow the post-psychotic regression to continue until Phase III appears.)

Marked differences exist with respect to where to focus the content of early interviews—on the patient's past, the interaction with the therapist, or his adaptation; on the patient's aggression or sadness; and on realities or fantasies. A major controversy about technique is the relative emphasis given to relationship and exploration in producing change. The second major technique debate concerned the role of regression in treatment—how much to permit it and when to attempt to prevent it. Finally, there was disagreement as to whether to conceptualize the schizophrenic's basic failure to manage the threatened loss of a sustaining object in terms of intolerable affect or unstable introjects and, in either case, whether this basic dysfunction is a deficit or defense.

The conclusions are drawn that there is a need for less provincialism and for more controlled studies on process variables. There remains much room for both schizophrenia research and schizophrenia psychotherapists to benefit from each other's experience. This may be needed if the psychotherapy of schizophrenia is to be influenced by research results and if the psychotherapy is to become more of a science than an art.

We have observed repeatedly that investigators approaching the problem of schizophrenia with nonclinical techniques have not defined the kind of subject they were studying. The question of what schizophrenia is has not been adequately answered. Any program of research on schizophrenia should inevitably reach a working definition of the category as a whole and of its subgroups. At present, we understand schizophrenia to be characterized by disorders of thinking, feeling, and sensory-motor function.

Arieti's description of four longitudinal stages is helpful.

Arieti's Longitudinal Stages (1955)

1. *Initial Stage:* Intense anxiety and panic with a sense of strangeness that might alternate with psychotic insight, accompanied by the feeling of being exceptionally lucid:
   a. If catatonic, overwhelmed by fear of actions;
   b. If hebephrebic, swayed by unconscious forces that implicate paleological thinking;
   c. If paranoid, remaining conscious with logical forces mobilized in the service of the unconscious; that is, logical forces are used to corroborate and sustain feelings and ideas that are emotionally determined and paleologically conceived.
2. *Advanced Stage:* Anxiety is no longer observed; suffering from delusions and hallucinations is diminished; and less active and more stereotyped behavior is associated with desocializing process.
3. *Preterminal Stage:* This occurs from five to fifteen years after onset, but may occur sooner or later; hallucinations and delusions have disappeared; hoarding and self-decorative habits are prominent.
4. *Terminal Stage:* Some of the symptoms, e.g. increased oral preoccupations and activities, are neurological symptoms, rather than psychological. ("The indefinite quality of some of the symptoms leaves ample space for speculation and makes their study difficult.")

Some years ago, Apter (1959) of our group described the behavioral changes that occur in chronic schizophrenic patients from the deepest regressive states to remission, of longer or shorter duration, of the psychosis. These findings are now summarized as a source of comparison with the phasic changes Kayton has described in acute psychoses. The patients in Apter's study who achieve Grade I and II levels are regarded as "irreversible." Attainment of clinical states from Grade III to Grade IV warrants a classification as "reversible." These grades are defined as follows.

Grade I: The first shift in behavior occurs as a change in motility patterns. Peculiar posturing; fixed facial expressions; and bizarre, automatic associated movements disappear. Relaxation of the facial musculature and loosening of motor activity in large and small joints are the initial signs of remission.

Grade II: Spontaneous activity increases and is associated with continued flexibility of motor patterns. Previously untidy and incontinent patients begin to take care of their own housekeeping functions.

Grade III: The spontaneous activity is extended to meet some of the socializing goals of the ward. Verbal communication is at a minimum or absent. In this phase, the predominantly catatonic patients remain nonverbal but volunteer to participate in group functions and give evidence of a feeling of belonging by assuming responsibilities for the group.

Group IV: Freer communication on both motor and verbal levels is exhibited, with some willingness to reach out for interpersonal contacts.

Inquiries concerning relatives are made. Letter writing occasionally occurs. Affective discharges are more common. The previously passive, docile patient may give expression to aggressive behavior. Patients with predominantly paranoid features begin to exhibit aspects of their premorbid personality. In them, hostility, suspiciousness, and combative attitudes are replaced by oversolicitousness, docility, submissiveness, and superficial cooperativeness. The greater majority of chronic schizophrenic patients do not progress beyond this stage.

Grade V: An improvement in the clinical picture appears in terms of ability to socialize, communicate past and current feelings, recall important relationships, meet with relatives, and display more or less appropriate affective responses. There remains, however, marked fragility of relationships, feelings of confusions, lack of identity, and evasiveness about leading emotional conflicts.

Grade VI: This appears as a temporary remission. There is a dissolution of the bizarre symptomatology with generalized planning for resumption of life outside the hospital. In one instance, a willingness to deal with major emotional conflicts and the events leading up to the catastrophic reaction appeared. This patient communicated his deep insights into the precipitating events and their meanings in relation to his illness.

The most recent paper published by our schizophrenic research group discusses the relationship between anhedonia and schizophrenia (Harrow et al., 1977) :

> The authors administered semi-structured interviews to 187 psychiatric inpatients to determine the role of anhedonia in schizophrenia. The interviews were tape-recorded and then given blind ratings for anhedonia on a 7-point scale. Schizophrenic patients had significantly more anhedonic tendencies. Most of the difference between the groups resulted from high anhedonia scores for chronic schizophrenics; less anhedonia was found in the acute schizophrenic patients. The data indicate that anhedonia is not necessary or unique to schizophrenia but is a prominent factor in chronic schizophrenia.

Since depression as well as periods of elation occur in schizophrenics, many are diagnosed as manic-depressives, especially by the British, who traditionally minimize the aspect of thought disorder. Conversely, American clinicians concentrate on the latter and resolve the combinations of affective and disturbed thinking by hedging, by diagnosing these patients as schizoaffective schizophrenics. Some patients clearly do not belong in this category, and their ultimate diagnosis cannot be determined by less than a long-term longitudinal study. The elation in these patients usually is not amenable to lithium, and the depression does not respond to the tricyclic drugs. The affective component, as an indicator of a good prognosis, is controversial.

The P & PI Schizophrenic Research Program

The basic *method* was the clinical study and taped interviews of a random sample of patients between 18 and 28 who were admitted to the hospital, and gave informed consent (confidentiality was assured), and who agreed to continue cooperating in further studies. Taped interviews conducted by Roy R. Grinker, Sr., and other trained clinicians, were rated with our Schizophrenic Trait Inventory (SSI), coded and punched on cards suitable for further statistical studies, including correlations, factor analysis, discriminate functional studies, and other multivariate statistics. We planned to interview *500 subjects and follow them annually to age 40.*

The sample of patients planned for this study involved schizophrenic and nonschizophrenic patients between 18 and 29 years of age. The schizophrenic sample included the following subdiagnostic breakdown: schizoaffective patients, acute schizophrenics, chronic schizophrenics, acute-chronic schizophrenics (chronic schizophrenics with a sharp, acute break), and paranoid schizophrenics.

The nonschizophrenic patients (a parallel sample between 18 and 28 years of age, hospitalized at the same inpatient setting) consisted of affective disorders (both unipolar and bipolar), personality disorders, neurotic disorders, patients with anorexia nervosa, borderline syndrome, narcissistic patients, and patients with organic syndromes. A number of substudies of these nonschizophrenic patient groups were conducted by our research team to determine the relationship between these nonschizophrenic groups and schizophrenia, and the theoretical significance of the overlapping clinical and nonclinical features.

The research encompassed patient interviews, clinical observations and tests, and studies of the patients' parents and siblings. Thus, in addition to the study of the patients via the patient interviews and other data collection methods during the acute phase, the major coordinating projects which are providing valuable data and which use the same basic sample of patients were as follows:

1) Studies of information processing with a particular emphasis on possible memory disorders as an influence on schizophrenic cognition, by Soon Duk Koh.
2) Follow-up studies encompassing research on cognition, outcome, and prognosis, being conducted by Martin Harrow.
3) Family studies by Froma Walsh.
4) Studies of disordered thinking by Martin Harrow.
5) Studies of chronic reversible and irreversible subjects by Nathaniel Apter.
6) Studies involving repeated interviews of the patient sample at subsequent admission to the hospital, by Roy R. Grinker, Sr., and other trained interviewers.

Although it was not our intention during the planning stage, our design leads us to study and compare all psychiatric diseases and disturbances in living.

The above summary presents some of our research strategy and findings from our past experiments. Although the schizophrenic deficit appears to be everywhere according to the literature, our studies thus far lead us to believe that (a) the schizophrenics' knowledge of the world, lexical representation, and strategic repertoire are probably not impaired, that (b) they are simply inefficient in spontaneously utilizing these adequate internal resources in their performance (a production deficiency), and that (c) their performance in remembering can be remedied by experimentally enhancing the mnemonic strategies. We are even tempted to speculate that the dysfunction of the schizophrenics' executive control is similar to the clinical notion of the ego dysfunction in schizophrenia. The major difference, however, lies in the fact that the theoretical constructs can be studied in the information-processing approach by both independent but converging experiments and their partial replications. These constructs which are objectively identified, isolated, and validated would, therefore, greatly reduce the usual gaps between the theory and data, and consequently, more concretely contribute to our effort to theorize about the schizophrenic psychopathology, to assess the drug effects, and to ameliorate the schizophrenic difficulties in mnemonic processing.

Findings which distinguished families of schizophrenics *(S)* from disturbed *(D)* and normal *(N)* control groups:

Relationship Patterns (Summers and Walsh, 1977; Walsh, in press)

(1) *Diadic relationships:* Mother-child, father-child, and mother-father relationships were assessed on rating scales developed for mother, father, and child interviews and projective stories, on three dimensions hypothesized by earlier investigators as important in schizophrenia: (Subjects: $S = 17, D = 14, N = 15$)

a. *Symbiosis:* Specific to the schizophrenic group, the mother-child relationship was found to be characterized by a symbiotic bond. The schizophrenic child showed stronger dependency than did the index child in control groups. Most interestingly, the *mother's need for the bond for her own well-being* was a more significant factor than was concern for the well-being of the child.
b. *Disconfirmation:* The father-child bond in the schizophrenic group was uniquely characterized by father's tendency to disconfirm the child and yet to interfere with his (her) life.
c. *Marital Dissatisfaction:* A significantly higher rate of marital relationships in the schizophrenic group were found to be unsatisfactory to both parents.
d. *Grandparents Death As Critical Stress Event:* The above finding led to further analysis of occurrence of grandparent

deaths at critical times in the lives of parents and index child finding:

1. In 45% of schizophrenic cases ($N = 55$) a grandparent died within two years of the birth of the schizophrenic child, a frequency significantly higher than both control groups ($p = < .01$)
   a. In 6 cases where a schizophrenic patient had a non-schizophrenic hospitalized sibling also in the study, all six schizophrenics had a grandparent death occur around this birth while this did not occur for any of the six disturbed but non-schizophrenic siblings.
   b. The deaths were equally distributed through pregnancy and infancy.
   c. No other four year time period showed such a high frequency of grandparent deaths for any of the three groups.
   d. Maternal grandparent deaths were no more frequent than paternal, and grandmother deaths no more frequent than grandfather. Same-sex vs. opposite sex comparisons yielded no significant differences.
2. For 30% of the schizophrenics, the patient age at onset of illness corresponded to the exact age of one parent at the death of his (her) parent.

Overall, the results from our research project question standard ideas about disordered thinking, and fundamental and primary symptoms of schizophrenia. To summarize our findings in this area, bearing on concepts about thought pathology as primary symptoms of schizophrenia, our approach via longitudinal investigations appear to indicate that:

1. Disordered thinking is more common, but not unique, to schizophrenia.
2. Disordered thinking is not clearly predictive of outcome in schizophrenia.
3. Disordered thinking does not persist in all types of schizophrenia.
4. Disordered thinking does not appear to be an index of the severity of the schizophrenic disorder.

Overall, our results in this area suggest that while thought pathology does play an important role in schizophrenia, it can be seriously questioned whether disordered thinking fits traditional ideas about "primary" symptoms in schizophrenia.

Some of the results which have emerged are listed below:

1. Schizophrenics functioned more poorly than non-schizophrenics during the follow-up period despite extensive use of phenothia-

zines and psychotherapy. ($p < .001$). (In the Methods section of this grant proposal we have discussed the issue of medication and its influence on functioning at greater length).

2. A core group of schizophrenics (almost 50%) were functioning very poorly in at least two of the three major areas at follow-up.
3. 62% of the schizophrenics were rehospitalized at least once.
4. The young paranoid and chronic schizophrenics tended to have higher rates of rehospitalization and poorer functioning than the schizo-affective and acute schizophrenics.
5. The poorer posthospital functioning of the schizophrenics was not limited to psychotic symptoms and social deterioration, but cut across all areas of adjustment.
6. The data suggests that our modern treatment techniques are not as effective with certain core groups of severe outcome schizophrenics.
7. It may be the large group of *intermediate outcome schizophrenics* who profit more from modern treatment techniques. These intermediate outcome schizophrenics now experience mild, and sometimes severe, difficulties in functioning, and sporadic rehospitalization, rather than severe deterioration and years of chronic hospitalization.
8. The results do not agree with casual observations that after treatment ⅓ of schizophrenics function well, ⅓ function equivocally, and ⅓ function poorly.
9. Only 15-20% of the schizophrenics were later functioning at a high level without relapses, a result not much superior to that in the Bleuler-Kraepelin era, 60-75 years ago.

Overall, along with a series of other findings about outcome, the early results suggest that modern day schizophrenics do function better after hospitalization than during the Kraepelin-Bleuler era. However, our data suggests that as a group they still have a relatively unfavorable outcome.

Shanfield et al. (1970) give an apt summary of schizophrenic symptomology that is an appropriate conclusion to this chapter:

In general, it seems logical to view depressive symptoms as an important part of the symptom complex for some schizophrenic patients. Clinicians tend to organize observations around abstract conceptualizations of symptom patterns called syndromes and, as such, these preconceptions may color our perception of various symptoms. Behavior which may appear or may be labeled as retarded, withdrawn, and isolated in the depressed patient, may be described as apathetic, affectless, and autistic when seen in a schizophrenic patient. It is clear from these data that depressive symptoms are an important part of the presenting picture of some schizophrenic patients. As such, they are fequently overlooked, but they also may be of a differnt quality (some have characterized this state in schizophrenics as wooden appearance; empty) and quantity than depressive symptomatology in the classical depressed patient. An awareness of the presence of these depressive symptoms and how they change over time is important for the treatment and understanding of the schizophrenic patient.

CHAPTER 11

Borderline States

DURING THE LAST SEVERAL DECADES, I have observed that the various psychiatric entities have changed considerably. There are fewer dramatic or histrionic neuroses, and the psychotics have become less florid and dangerous. There have been more constricted and restricted characters. These seemed to conform to what has been called the *borderline syndrome.*

It is difficult to determine when the term *borderline* was first used and by whom. However, from 1884 *borderline* or *borderland* has designated conditions between schizophrenic and neuroses of various kinds. Often, the diagnosis for some seemed to indicate a latent, potential, or transitional phase of schizophrenia.

Schmideberg (1959) applied the descripton of "stable instability" to the borderline, since normality, neuroses, psychoses, and psychopathy blended in a lifelong pattern. These patients do not have a characteristic symptom pattern, but unhappily have weak object relations.

From the literature on the borderline, we are convinced that there is scarcely a general understanding of the term and no consensus on differentiating criteria that would lead to accurate, consistent, and reliable diagnoses. There are few clinical descriptive or psychoanalytic reports based on supportive data, and there are only confused dynamic formulations. Several central ideas run through the concepts and images that clinicians hold of these patients. They generally agree that borderline patients look clinically unclear and that they occupy an area in psychopathology where accurate diagnosis is difficult. Beyond this small island of common ground, varying assumptions are made.

There is a variety of clinical positions. Some say there is no such thing as borderline, that patients are schizophrenics; others say that the borderline may be a transitional state from neurosis to psychosis; and finally others believe that the borderline is a relatively stable personality disturbance with psychotic, neurotic, and health ego-functions present simultaneously, and that the range of symptoms includes those characteristic of an extensive spectrum from neurotic to psychotic. Whichever of the last two positions is taken, there is agreement that among these patients certain ego-functions are rather severely impaired.

This, then, is the problem as derived from experiences in practice with patients who were unclearly defined and usually unsuccessfully treated. Is the term *borderline* a wastebasket into which all puzzling cases are dumped? Are there clinical, dynamic, or other characteristics that could define them as members of a single nosological category, and are there multiple subcategories?

From another point of view, Knight (1954) described weak or impaired ego-functions in the borderline. Likewise, Kernberg (1967) describes a lack of stable ego-identity because of conflictual identifications. It must be emphasized that all these authors and others consider that the borderline represents a defect in psychological development and not a regression.

In an effort to determine the characteristics of the borderline category and its subcategories if any, Werble, and Drye (1968) carried out a lengthy and complicated clinical investigation. We admitted to a hospital unit young adults with uncertain diagnoses who had intact cognitive functioning, appropriate associations, and no systematized delusions or paranoid attitudes. Some had brief histrionic psychotic attacks between which there was good psychological functioning. In sum, the precipitating causes for hospitalizations were (1) depressive loneliness with suicidal ideation or attempts; (2) impulsive angry eruptions; (3) alcoholism, compulsions, and phobias, and (4) temporary confusional states.

The subjects were closely observed over each twenty-four-hour period for two weeks after adjustment to hospitalization (about two weeks). The observations were made by personnel who served the patients: nurses, attendants, and activities and occupational workers. The observations included attention to verbal and nonverbal behaviors.

The observers then described the subjects' behaviors to an interviewer who had not seen or come in contact with them. The report was taped and transcribed and included anywhere from fifteen to twenty descriptions by various observers during all shifts in the two-week period.

Analyses of transcribed reports were made according to five major attributes of ego-functions derived from ninety-three well-defined variables. The attributes were (1) outward behavior, adaptation to people, environment, and tasks; (2) perception and sense of reality; (3) language capacity; (4) affects and defenses; and (5) problem solving and global organization.

Using statistical clustering, discriminate and factor analyses revealed that the borderline patient in general has a defect in his affectional relationships, occasional angry explosions, lack of consistent self-identity, and depression characterized by loneliness rather than guilt or shame.

Within this general category, there were four subcategories. *Group I* were inappropriate and negative in their relations to others and were often given to impulsive angry outbursts, sometimes so overwhelming ego-controls so that they became temporarily psychotic for an hour, a day, or a week but rarely more. They had a deficient sense of self and were often depressed.

Group II showed vacillating involvement with others, moving toward and quickly away from object-relations—back and forth like a yo-yo. *Group III* showed adaptive and appropriate behavior achieved by an "as if" kind of posture, little spontaneity, and evidences of defensive withdrawal *Group IV* had more anxiety and a childlike, clinging depression.

Though there was a good deal of overlapping within the subcategories, enough differences could be discriminated within the characteristics of the general category to permit a specific diagnosis.

In 1970, Gruenewald performed an extensive battery of psychological tests on ten borderline subjects. These tests supported the diagnosis on all essential points and confirmed the characteristics of the subgroups for the syndrome. There was no movement from one subgroup to another. Structural defects of the ego were present and there was evidence of early disturbances in relations of objects and tenuous impulse control.

Previously, the differential diagnosis of the borderline had not been attempted. The syndrome had been seen as symptomatic of a latent schizophrenia, depression, or personality and character disorder. The defensive symptoms *over and above the essential core process* were thought to represent neurotic, personality, and delinquent overlaps, including alcoholism, drug abuse, sexual promiscuity, and perversions.

It is clear, however, that the borderline does not have the thought disorders characteristic of even latent schizophrenia. He does not have the capacity to develop schizophrenia, as does the pseudoneurotic schizophrenic. Group I, sometimes termed *psychotic characters,* have only brief periods of disorganization associated with rage attacks. Disturbances in associations, autistic thinking, defects in language and logical thought and delusions or hallucinations are not included in the personality of the borderline. In fact, he is suffering from a disease *sui generis.*

In summary, the borderline syndrome is prepared by some unknown *developmental variants.* The early mother-infant transactions are usually blamed for this and other disturbances, but there is no sound proof for such an assumption. The borderline personality is a life-style of vacillating eccentricity. What pushes it into the overt syndrome or back into a remission is not known.

Like those of most other psychiatric disturbances, the etiology of the borderline cannot be pinpointed either from a specific or a systems approach. All that can be said is that "the borderline, like health and illness is a system in process occurring in time: developing, progressing and regressing as a focus in a large biopsychosocial field." The biogenetic, experiential, psychological, and social parts of the system are unknown. Yet, the borderline is increasing in numbers, as are other neuroses and psychoses of restricted and constricted personalities. Reports published in the foreign literature, as well as in this country, indicate that the borderline syndrome may appear in childhood and in chronic lifelong psychiatric patients, suggesting as does all the other evidence that the syndrome represents a defect in development.

Perry and Klerman (1968) state that the

> research reported by Grinker and his associates merits high praise for a number of reasons. First, it builds upon previous work. Their review of the literature is comprehensive and sophisticated. Second, the research is empirical and systematic. They studied a series of patients ($N = 51$), moderate in size in comparison to the literature of usual research in psychopathology but enormous in size by comparison to the literature on the borderline patient. Third, they used advanced methods of quantitative rating scales and multivariate statistical analysis. Fourth, they delineated four sub-types by cluster analysis and related the sub-types to clinical experience. And fifth, they have attempted to validate their typology by follow-up study and by correlations with family dynamics.

After we (Grinker, Werble, and Drye) published our research monograph on the borderline in 1968 after eight years of work observing, describing, rating and statistical analysis, we were satisfied that we had described a separate entity with four subtypes. But such research that isolates a syndrome sacrifices detailed protocols of individual patients. We attempted to rectify this by reporting in some detail a few descriptions of individual patients. Apparently these were not sufficient nor clear enough, because clinicians had difficulty in diagnosing their own patients.

Two major mistakes are constantly reported at meetings and in publications. The first is the use of the term *borderline schizophrenia.* Our work and that of others indicates that the schizophrenias exist as syndromes characterized by specific behaviors, affects, and thought disorders. A person is either schizophrenic or he is not. Schizophrenia is not latent or borderline. Furthermore, schizophrenia is not equivalent to psychoses. This term applies to schizophrenics who have disintegrated; to some manic-depressives; and to psychoses related to toxins, infections, trauma, cerebral arteriosclerosis, and senility. A person may be close to a psychotic break, but his essential problem is not the final psychotic disintegration, which occurs in about 40 percent of the pseudoneurotic schizophrenias described by Hoch and Polatin (1959).

Second, the diagnosis of the borderline schizophrenia is based on a series of *core phenomena* consisting of developmental or distortions of ego-functions. These are anger as the main or only affect, a defect in attaining and maintaining affectional relationships, an absence of adequate self-identity, and depressive loneliness. The four subtypes deal with such defects in a variety of ways, but these defenses, substitutions, and adaptations do not constitute the borderline and are no different from those seen in a variety of other psychiatric disturbances. These *secondary neurotic and behavioral symptoms* include fantasy, religious preoccupation, drug addiction and abuse, alcoholism, anorexia or obesity, or suicide attempts and a wide variety of other secondary symptoms *overlying the essence of the borderline.*

In a later study, we described the stress responses of a group of ten middle-aged, male subjects who manifested chronic and intractable psychiatric illness. The group represented a nosological category best described as "inadequate," but all had depression as their presenting symptom. Historical and behavioral data revealed that our subjects had a characteristic pervasive tendency to avoid and shut out all stressful stimuli. Thus, they seem unaffected by external disturbance. Maneuvers consonant with this stood out in their behavior during the stress interview. Despite their energetic efforts to shut this out, too, the interviewer was successful in producing a meaningful breakthrough because he was able to disrupt their status quo while simultaneously obstructing all avenues of escape. Despite the general nonresponsiveness, the interview produced a stress response as indicated by emotional arousal, increases in heart rate and blood pressure, and adrenocortical stimulation (Oken, 1962).

Since we had previously studied the response of acutely ill psychiatric patients to a similar stimulus, control data were available for comparison. The responses of the present subjects were distinctive in that they were sharply delimited to the stress period, whereas the acute group came to the situation already somewhat aroused and manifested a response that persisted beyond the nuclear stress. The focal nature of the observed response is quite compatible with the characteristics of the defensive structure described. Apparently, there is no interference with the capacity to respond, but rather an extraordinarily efficient exclusion of stimuli that might excite response. This hyperconstricted type of defensive organization represents an open and overgeneralized responses of the acute group and is equally seriously maladaptive.

It is suggested that this type of psychosomatic organization may be one characteristic of what is termed the *chronic borderline state.*

As a result of careful study of 14 new borderline cases made available through current research, we have been able to add the following observations. Of 14 patients, 9 were rated high on anhedonia (lacked early experiences of pleasure) ; 10 were rated high on depression and/or anger; 12 dated the onset of their problems to childhood; 12 had school problems, often being expelled or dropping out; 10 reported suicidal thoughts or attempts; 11 were rated high on identity problems; 10 showed emotional attachments to their family or surrogates (dependency) ; 10 were rated as having little or no affection for peer group or nonfamily members; 9 were rated as confused; and all 14 were rated as lacking organization. There have been a number of additional observations. The first, on the basis of family studies, is that anorexia nervosa in these patients seems to be a means of indirectly expressing anger at the family.

Two additional empirical findings with respect to the family of origin for borderline patients revealed that in ten of the fourteen cases there was a family history of mental problems of various types. Also, a much higher incidence of divorce and parent loss was observed in this group than in a comparison group of schizophrenics. Aspects of this information are summarized:

Families	*Borderline Patients (%)*	*Schizophrenics (%)*
Intact	42.9	75.6
Divorce in family	35.7	15.4
Parent death	21.4	9.0

By contrasting borderline patients with schizophrenic patients in the present research program, it has been found that the borderline differs from the schizophrenic in several significant ways. Unlike the schizophrenic, the borderline does not exhibit:

1. Disturbances in intellectual associational processes
2. Autistic or regressive thinking
3. Family characteristics of "pseudomutuality" or "skewing"
4. Delusions or hallucinations

5. Deficit in connotative aspects of language

In addition, we have recently reported that the character of psychotic (or psychoticlike) behavior, when it does occur, is different from that observed in schizophrenic psychoses. In particular, psychotic episodes in borderlines seem to be induced by quantities of rage unmanageable by the deficient defensive functions of the ego.

As a result of the data from our coordinated studies, we have begun to elaborate and qualify the character of depression in the borderline patient by contrasting it with depression in patients given this latter single diagnosis. Thus, we have recently observed that "in general, it can be stated that, although depression as an affect is found in several of the borderline categories, it does not correspond with that seen in the depressive syndrome (Grinker and Werble, 1977).

Behaviors we observed while researching delineated disturbances of ego-functions of the borderline and were statistically analyzed into groups and factors. The resultant scientific skeleton requires the flesh and blood of recognizable symptoms to become useful for clinicians.

The syndrome or borderline class of patients has difficulty in achieving and maintaining affectional relations; they have trouble in controlling aggressive impulses and rarely achieve a consistent reliable and satisfying identity. Ego-alien, short-lived confusional, or paranoidlike psychoses may occur, as well as temporary states of loneliness, appearing as depression without guilt and depression of the anaclitic clinging type. Absent are evidences of cognitive disturbances, looseness of associations, or hallucinations or delusions, as seen in the following case reports.

Case 1

At the time of admission to the P & PI, the patient was a thirty-year-old mother of two who was separated from her husband. She had been living with her parents while her children were in the custody of her husband in California. On admission, she was confused as to the reasons for admission, saying, "I don't know whether I should be here or not. My father wanted me to come." In this way she disclaimed responsibility for her treatment but would accept the facilities of the hospital, ultimately taking advantage of the hospital for room, board, and social life.

Anamnesis revealed that her difficulties had begun some four years previously. On the surface, she had been doing well with her husband and two children. However, she resented his seeming lack of interest in her sexually; he had taken a job as a traveling salesman, which kept him away from her a good deal of the time. As her resentment increased, she accepted a dinner invitation from friends *she knew her husband would resent.* For the entire day before the dinner and while at the dinner she felt an aimless dread but had no insight as to why she should feel so upset. Nothing unusual occurred, however, and she returned home, going to bed without incident. Early the next morning, however, she was awakened by pain in her left shoulder radiating down the arm to the fingers, associated with difficulty in breathing. She feared she would die, awakened her husband and was rushed to an emergency room where she was told that she only had "nerve trouble" and needed some counseling.

For the next two years, the patient received intensive psychotherapy from a male psychiatrist who saw her three times a week, ultimately decreasing to once a week. At one point during her therapy she became "suicidal," and although she had made no suicidal attempt, she was hospitalized for three months, being allowed to sign out then against medical advice. Toward the end of the therapy, she developed strong erotic feelings for her psychiatrist, characterized by sexual daydreams, dressing in a seductive way for her sessions, and beginning an affair with a neighbor. At about this time, her husband became more attentive to her. She felt things were going well and terminated the treatment, although the psychiatrist felt she needed more. For four months, she felt relatively well, but when her lover moved to another part of the state, depression set in. She sought further psychiatric care from a second male psychiatrist who concurred with her own desire for electric shock treatment.

Following the second course of treatment, she told her husband of her recent affair, and the marital relationship deteriorated. He began to drink, she began to drink and use drugs, and soon they separated. Periodically she would be visited by her lover, and during such times she would feel well, but at other times she was quite depressed. Her ability to take care of the home and children deteriorated. One year before admission to a hospital her elder child was hit by a car and suffered a brain concussion. Following the child's recovery, she granted her husband a divorce, took a second lover, and became depressed after he asked her to marry him. Six months before admission, she took an overdose of sleeping pills, planned so that her lover found her unconscious, and she was hospitalized for a second time. While she was hospitalized, the court granted custody of the children to her husband, and upon discharge the patient moved in with a girl friend. At that time, she was unable to do more than drink and be isolated in the house.

The patient's family then persuaded her to return home, where she saw a psychiatrist once a week but remained isolated in her parents' apartment. Because of increasingly severe depression and drinking, her parents forced her psychiatrist to place her in a hospital where she stayed for one month. Almost immediately upon admission, the depression dissipated, and she began to function with the patient group as if she had been a long-standing member. She had two affairs while in the hospital—one with an attendant and one with a nurse from another hospital. All in all, she felt more relaxed and more comfortable in the hospital than ever before. Because of her improvement, she was discharged; once home with her parents, interminable arguments and drinking began. After an argument she took some pills, slashed her wrists superficially, and was readmitted to the hospital.

The patient was born and raised in Chicago. She is the elder of two children, with a brother six years younger. When asked about her early life, she remembered that when she was about three or four her parents lived near her grandmother's home but *she was always left out of the communication between her mother, father, and grandparents.* While her parents were always "terribly devoted to each other," she felt, *"I never belonged. Maybe that is why I felt a wall around me. I can't feel."* Although she said she was always "mother's and daddy's little girl who never wanted for anything because of the type of family I lived in," in the next breath she would say *she was always unsure of herself.*

In high school, when she was elected secretary of the senior class, she noticed that the other girls who were elected officers seemed to be experiencing strong emotions, including crying and exuberance, while *she herself could feel nothing. In fact, she reported that she could not feel anything except when she took drugs.*

The patient is aware of how angry she sometimes becomes and how her angry outbursts often jeopardize her relationships. One such example occurred in elementary school. The patient's mother said to her one day that, if it was 40 degrees outside the next day, the patient wouldn't have to wear leggings. The patient was pleased, because that meant she might not have to wear the hated clothes. The following morning, mother said that the patient had to wear her leggings. The patient became angry and decided to leave home to go to her grandmother's house. She remembered walking very slowly because she was frightened, and she kept looking back over her shoulder, hoping that someone would come after her.

"This is kind of what I do when I make suicidal attempts, hoping someone will save me. Finally my father did overtake me and took me home. I was glad. I was really quite relieved. When I was in California recently I told my folks over the phone that I felt like killing myself, that they did this to me. I also called my mother to tell her that I'd kill myself but what could she do about it. I guess I just wanted to hurt her. And I told my husband about the affair to shock and hurt him, and tell him how bad I really was. *I guess I've always done things to be cruel, to hurt other people.*"

The patient dated a neighbor's son, T., for a couple of years while in high school. Finally, she broke up with T. and started dating W. and D. Subsequently, T. asked her out again, and instead of refusing as her other girl friends had encouraged her to do, she went out with him immediately. For a period of several years, she dated T., W., and D. interchangeably. *She did not have a preference except for the boy that she was with at the moment.*

This patient represents a prototype of Group I of the borderline. In her own statement she has never considered that she "belonged" and says very clearly that she cannot feel. Her early role assignment was that of an object of mother's narcissism; mother's concerns were of appearance and behavior, not of feelings. Having no help with her feelings, they were taken as signs of her badness, and *she developed a self-image of worthlessness.* When she attempted independence and self-reliance, she was inhibited by mother's controls.

Now she shows she is unsure of herself; *her self-image is that of an inferior person who must anxiously attempt to meet standards of others. She has difficulty in feeling anything except when she is comfortable in the hospital where there are relatively well-defined roles or when she is under the influence of alcohol or of drugs. In order to get a feeling of belonging and identity, the patient must attach herself to someone, living an almost parasitic relationship.* Information regarding her high school boyfriends indicates that she did not have a preference, except for *"the boy I was with at the moment."* Her elopement was an impulsive desire to hang on to someone. Inward attachments, in order to be of significance to her, in view of her lack of ability to experience feelings, *take the form of violent feelings, either hurting herself or hurting others.* Thus, her relation with others may be quite intense but is unstable. In this sense, she is like a tabetic who has to stamp the ground to feel; to feel, the relationship must be violent.

In a vain attempt to resolve her loneliness and need for attention, the patient gradually acquires the role of the sick person; her conversion symptoms, alcoholism, drug abuse, and hospitalization are the signs of this newly developed role.

Thus, we see a patient *unable to form stable affectionate relationships,* to control aggressive feelings, or to develop a coherent self-identity, vainly trying to escape from depression by promiscuity, drugs, alcohol, and hospitalization.

Case 2

A thirty-two-year-old female entered the hospital, *expressing anger* at the entire environment. She was so outspoken that negative reactions were evoked from everyone. Nevertheless, she had to have things her own way—right or wrong. At times she was so loud that she had to be controlled from inappropriate gales of laughter. When her husband called and left a message that her *sick daughter was feeling better, she evidenced no response and acted as if she had not heard.* Her appearance was that of a disheveled person who did not care about the environment, nor was she insulted when criticized. The patient was well aware of the time schedules of various activities, yet always shuffled in late. She monopolized group meetings with loud talk. She broke the rules concerned with proper dress and frequented the male section, which was off limits. *When intensely angry, she seemed to get farther and farther away from reality. There were no evidences of positive relations to anyone.*

Patients in Group I in general do not achieve a sense of consistent identity and have great difficulty in establishing positive relations with others. They apparently have given up actively trying to develop object-relations and withdraw more or less from the scene. *Yet, they are lonely, depressed, and enraged at the environment and other human beings.* It is this rage that has many behavioral outlets, but these are not sufficient to protect the *ego from transient and mild dissolution of the function of reality adaptation;* hence, the transient psychoses superimposed on inappropriate, nonadaptive, and negative behaviors.

Case 3

This twenty-two-year-old female was a school dropout, sometimes alcoholic, occasionally a drug user, promiscuous, and had one illegitimate pregnancy and abortion. Her psychotherapeutic sessions have been filled with accounts of vacillation between Joe and Larry, always breaking up with one or the other. *No evidence of any affectionate relationship was ever found, not even to a dog she bought and permitted to die,* and there were *no transference manifestations in the therapy.* "Well, I was mad all weekend. *I Just seemed to have so much hate.* I don't know what the hate was about but it was there. I seem to hate everybody. I certainly hate Joe and Larry and yet, I need them too."

I asked what she needed them for. She said, *"Well, I don't want to be alone. I'm just disgusted with the whole thing.* I don't really want to go back and yet I find that I am. It's like watching, waiting to see what I'm going to do next. It's almost like a play and *I have a certain role and I look to see what's going to happen in the next act.*

"I'm so disgusted, *I just feel that nobody cares!*"

"It seems that you would like to have closeness and concern and yet, when it's within my grasp there's something about it that seems to make me flee from it."

"Well, when you get into a relationship like that you get trapped. At first it's fine. But then you start getting in a pattern. You have to do what the other one wants you to do.

"It's like when I sleep with a boy for a few months. At first it's exciting and fun. And then after a while, I just have to keep going. Not 'cause I want to any more. Then I want to be free. I want to get out of the relationship, and I don't know how to do it. So then I have to start creating little incidents so that the other one will have to break up with me. I want my freedom then, but then, when I have my freedom, I just feel lonely again.

"The ideal relationship to me would be a two-month relationship. That way there'd be no commitment. At the end of the two months I could just break it off. The relationship would just evaporate and I'd be fine. But the only criterion for this would have to be someone else around so that I wouldn't get lonely."

In capsule form, this sector of a therapeutic session reveals all the characteristics of Group II: vacillating involvement with others; overt or acted-out expressions of anger; and varying degrees of lonely depressiveness and failure in achieving her own identity.

The patient received outpatient therapy for two years, but her pattern of desire and fear of closeness persisted. She was not committed to change and she developed no emotional insight, and by her own choice she stopped seeing the psychiatrist.

CHAPTER 12

Therapies, Service, and the Peer Groups

To say that there are varying goals of therapy is to express something of a paradox. In one sense, we have virtually the same goal: simply to improve or, if we dare say so, to cure our patients. In the past, one could identify an institution by the kinds of patients it admitted, the type of treatment it administered, and the length of stay it permitted. The number of variables was limited, waiting lists were enormous, and the time during which the patient had to suffer his disturbance outside of the private hospital was, accordingly, long.

By the twentieth century, the mentally ill were no longer considered to be witches or possessors of the devil. In the eighteenth century, the psychotic had been released from his chains and freed from bedlam, but his lot had improved very little. Many were incarcerated in overcrowded state hospitals, termed *warehouses,* and later, *snakepits.* Early in this century, neurotics were treated in psychiatrists' offices; the well-to-do psychotics in rest homes or sanitariums far from their families.

At present, the psychiatric hospital is all things to all patients, and there is rarely any sort of specialization. Most hospitals employ psychotherapy, milieu therapy, electric shock treatment, and occupational therapy, and there are a number of different kinds of centers for crisis intervention. Furthermore, the number of psychiatric units is increasing, and the number of such units that are attached to general hospitals, according to one survey, runs to about a thousand. By contrast, when I first started on the scene of a general hospital, I had only one model to imitate. Today, the larger and better psychiatric hospitals have training programs supported in whole or in part by the National Institute of Mental

Health. But, regardless of the source of support, only a broad range of patients and treatment procedures can adequately prepare the resident student to become a general psychiatrist. Most psychiatric hospitals also have research programs requiring the availability and use of a wide variety of case material. Today psychiatric hospitals and training centers are more alike than they are different.

The United States is a country of fashions that are largely imported. This fascination with imports is characteristic of psychiatry as well as of material goods. We have taken sleep treatment from Switzerland; insulin shock treatment from Austria; electric shock treatment from Italy; deconditioning from Russia; psychoanalysis from Austria; open– and day-hospital therapy from England; and occupational therapy from Germany, etc. We seem to have a tendency to accept these fashions with or without scientific evidence, and to incorporate them—for a time, at least.

Psychiatry no longer entertains the notion of cure, reconstruction of personality, or "adjustment." On the contrary, we help people in trouble to regain a stability that has been lost temporarily for a number of reasons, or we help them to attain a *degree* of adjustment which they have never had—in other words, to reestablish the continuity of development that has been interrupted at some time for a variety of reasons. We are often impressed by the fact that enthusiastic individuals appear on the scene from time to time with initial goals that astonish us. Frieda Fromm-Reichmann (1950), for example, felt at one time that she could cure schizophrenics. But, over the years, she modified her goals and was satisfied with much less. Many examples could be given. The older psychiatrists who have been through a variety of fashionable treatments are less enthusiastic, more realistic, and usually settle for far less. Perhaps this is the reason that we tend to give our hardest cases to the younger therapists.

Jerome Frank (1977) terms mental illness *demoralization* or shattered self-love, for which any treatment is better than waiting for spontaneous recovery. The goal of therapy is to help the subject learn to control his own life. To be effective, there must be a rationale that is convincing both to the patient and the therapist. The patient is required to participate actively and experience success through learning (behaviorism).

The differences in goals depend largely on temporal factors. Thus long- and short-term therapy have built-in goals that influence the kind of therapeutic procedure. For example, the emergency treatment that has been formalized by Jurgen Ruesch (1961) which maintains family contact, decreases the patient's dependency on the hospital, and attempts to get him rapidly back to his social milieu with continued therapy as an outpatient, is more feasible in urban centers where the outpatient department is available for ambulatory patients whose treatment can be continued by the same therapist. The availability of outpatient therapy, incidentally, should be of great importance in the choice of a hospital. The rapid discharge of patients after a short-term stay in a hospital accentuates the need for training in social skills, and for access to group therapy, milieu therapy, patient self-government, and day and night outpatient care.

The long-term residential therapies are applied to different types of patients who need individual psychotherapy or modified analysis and who are able to improve faster when removed from family and home to a separate environment. However, where there is difficulty in follow-up, the continuity of treatment is sorely interrupted. Some institutions are able to arrange for their patients to live after a time in foster homes and (particularly in the case of adolescents and children) in schools. What is important here is the recognition that therapy should mean what the patient needs and can use; it should not be based on stereotyped notions that derive from our own training orientations, curative ambitions, or personal biases. Sometimes the best course may be *to leave the patient alone.*

Therapy may take several forms: *pharmacotherapy* with phenothiazines, one of which is antischizophrenic and may prevent future psychoses with maintenance doses; psychotherapy; or various forms of sociotherapy within groups or within a favorable hospital milieu. The drug results seem most effective against a psychotic state. Though many anecdotes are available to prove the effectiveness of one method or another, we must emphasize here that hard statistics on results are not available. We can state that with the changing character of psychiatric diseases, and with the availability of antipsychotic drugs, the outlook for improvement and even recovery is increasing, and therapeutic optimism is justified. Furthermore, the decrease in the fear of schizophrenic rage and the increased ambulation of patients make long-term institutionalization far less necessary. I have had no experience with encounter groups, nor have they been conducted by my colleagues. But the "I scream," aggressive behavior, free sexuality, and touching, etc., groups are symptoms of an antipsychiatric attitude throughout the country. For the most part, they are commercial enterprises similar to the freaky oriental religions conducted by lay persons with no professional training or experience. No one engaged in them has been willing to subject his "methods" to scrutiny or follow up his clients to determine the results. However, Moos (1974) has described severe casualties resulting from them.

Military and civilian psychiatrists have learned that acute psychotic breakdowns are amenable to appropriate emergency "first aid" therapy. The faster the patient is found, the quicker the reestablishment of an equilibrium that may still carry with it the implications of "sickness," but not the dangers of his becoming a career hospitalized patient. However, as Jurgen Ruesch (1961) says, "It is easier to keep a patient than to treat him."

Ruesch recommends short-term hospitalization and early treatment with devices oriented to reestablishing ego controls, including psycho–, drug, and milieu therapy. The family's expectations for a speedy return of the patient should be encouraged. The patient should be led to anticipate rapid discharge. Immediate efforts should attempt to ascertain the triggering cue for his breakdown and ensure its removal or amelioration. The basic illness should be treated in the outpatient department after the patient has returned home and to work.

Strupp (1973) correctly states that analysts and many psychotherapists do not have their goals clearly in mind, or at least do not make explicit when they will expect to attain the highest possible level of improvement. The phenomenon of interminable treatment, which Alexander tried to combat with his concept or brief psychoanalysis (really psychotherapy), is common.

Results are difficult to evaluate for any therapy. What is good outcome and how long does it last? Wallerstein's (1966) report of the Menninger project indicated that even after hard, long, and tedious work the results were not conclusive, because of the many uncontrollable variables. Spiegel and I (1945), in our work on war neuroses, *Men Under Stress,* correctly predicted that, all along the line, from the combat zone to the continental United States, no matter what form of treatment, the results would be 60 to 70 percent improvement. One of our residents distributed a questionnaire to all of our therapists and their discharged patients from hospitals and clinics to compare the results of treatment among various mental health disciplines. Surprisingly, the patients reported a far better outcome than the therapists did. The latter had obviously held on to the illusion that character and personality could be reorganized, a feat which neither they or anyone else could achieve.

There is no substitute for long-term follow-up studies to verify diagnosis and to determine effectiveness of treatment. Despite devout statements, there is now no average expectable environment in which to receive treated patients—no ideal situation. The goal of health has to be related to the particular ethnic, social, and situational environment in which the subject works and lives. In addition, the behavioral characteristics of the psychiatric entities are changing. For example, there is currently less emphasis on conflict theory of the psychoses and more on developmental defects.

Just as psychoanalysts try to apply their special techniques to all patients, so do all therapists. Their loyalty to one technique does not last long, for the most part, though there is a reluctance to admit this. Training has been rigidly one-sided, and innovations are discouraged. As they get older, analysts become freer and more adaptive to the needs of their patients, rather than remaining bound to the theories they started with.

Strupp (1973) is correct when he advocates that investigations not be limited to practitioners who are members of a closed shop. To counteract our "inexact knowledge," he advocates more experiments, more empirical data, and a series of specifications or propositions for future research. These suggestions are highly commendable, but the tasks are difficult, and few competent people seem willing to undertake them. Perhaps Strupp is closer to reality when he states that "the future will not be utopia but neither need there be cause for despair."

It is as essential to determine what is common to all forms of psychotherapy as it is to determine what is specific to each. A few elements have special significance. The so-called therapeutic alliance is one of the most crucial. The patient is motivated to seek help to improve. He has faith that he can be helped. Such faith is strengthened by the therapist's respect and concern for the patient and his realistic expectations of what can be accomplished. But the therapist clearly needs auxiliary support.

Who knows what it is that actually helps the patient? One of our residents studied the African witch doctors, who spend two years in training. They house patients near their well-furnished, affluent houses, carry a bag of "instruments," speak in jargon, and charge high fees. The results are as good as any American therapist could accomplish!

Largely because of the number of uncontrolled variables—even when patients treated are compared with those on a waiting list—few people except Strupp have done statistical research on therapy itself. It is difficult to admit to my residents that there are no hard data on therapeutic research. I attempt to neutralize the blow by telling these young psychiatric missionaries that they will each build up a cachet of valid anecdotes based on their personal experiences, but that these will be specific to them and usually not generalizable or transferable. When they treat patients, at least those whom they do not dislike, they will be able to draw on their memory banks to insure that procedures that have been successful in the past will be carried out. But strict prescriptions as to what to say and when to say it, or the fear of inexact interpretations, need not worry them.

The most fundamental elements in psychoanalytic technique, ignoring the confused body of Freudian theory, are the regressive transference relationship and the interpretation of dreams. However, as Glover (1973) has stated, here, too; there are serious questions: "Psychoanalysts maintain an unrestricted license to interpret, which results in a degree of fabrication that validates their conclusions." Indeed, there is grave doubt that the transference can repeat infantile nonverbal childhood experiences.

Psychiatric treatment may take many forms. Psychotherapy can be based on a number of different techniques and theories, depending on the patient's needs and the therapist's ability. But support, direction, suggestion, and persuasion seem to be consistent elements, and these are present, to varying degrees, in the ancient techniques of hypnosis, as well as in the newer forms of behavior therapy for the neuroses. Individual therapy is always time consuming and expensive.

Group therapy is suitable for some patients. Participants tend to support one another, and group experiences enhance their social abilities and often ensure that they will take their medication. Some psychiatrists believe that group psychotherapy shortens overall hospitalization and there is some evidence that improvement is far greater than in individual therapy.

Although many psychiatrists have the idea that patients from low socioeconomic groups are not suitable for psychotherapy, this is not true. It is true, however, that relatively unsophisticated patients are more apt to expect instant results and are in a hurry (for obvious reasons) to leave the hospital and return to job and/or home. Once they are gone, it is extremely difficult to persuade them to continue treatment on an outpatient basis.

An altogether different social form of therapy is based on the philosophy of Kierkegaard. The *existential psychiatrist* attempts to help his patients who are afraid of not being free to find themselves in ways that do not dichotomize them and that make sense in the social, economic world in which they live. What is emphasized is that such persons can be free selves only as part of the society in which they live—not through hallucinatory drugs or by living in isolated communities.

Another group of psychiatrists, who may be called *sociotherapists,* emphasize milieu therapy in the hospital or practice group or family therapy for in– and outpatients. More than the others, this group veers away from the medical model, not only in the treatment modality, but also in their denigration of diagnostic terms and specific therapies. They repudiate the concept of mental illness, substituting for it "disturbances resulting from problem living." Society has in part accepted this distinction, as

I have already pointed out. The "encounter groups" that have proliferated dismay many of us. They are less expensive and require less of a time commitment, but their effectiveness has not been proven. They have led to fraudulent organizations, untrained leaders, and emotional casualties. Patients must be cautious about joining such enterprises.

Somatotherapists adhere to the medical model, using electric shock whenever possible and depending on a wide range of drugs, including the antischizophrenic and antidepressive drugs, including lithium (for manic attacks), either singly or in combination. Psychotherapists are increasingly willing to use drugs as adjuncts and facilitators of their own brand of therapy. Although previously doctors and nurses were biased against the use of drugs, there is currently a positive bias toward the value of medication, so much so in fact that it is hard to find unmedicated patients to use in the evaluation of specific forms of treatment.

In the last two decades, there has been a shift from considering psychoses self-limiting and from treating patients with bromides, phenobarbital, and opium, along with moral platitudes, to active psychopharmacology. Specific drugs are now available to counteract depressions, mania, anxieties, and psychoses; all of these drugs especially lithium must be carefully controlled. The side-effects must be countered and maintenance doses well calculated. For some psychotic depressives reacting poorly to medication, electroconvulsive therapy may be necessary, although it still carries with it some dangers.

The technical sequences used for involving a schizophrenic person in psychotherapy are complex and variable. Extended contact with a nonobtrusive but enthusiastic therapist who is full of curiosity about the patient is the basis for a corrective emotional experience that activates the hope that is required for reentry into close relationships. When these steps have been successfully taken, the previously reluctant patient may enter voluntarily into a psychotherapeutic program with some anticipation of success. Our findings about schizophrenia—its etiology and treatment—are treated in some depth in Chapter 10.

The treatment models that have been described correspond to the definition of psychiatry as a medical specialty devoted to the diagnosis and treatment of mental illness. The sharpness of the separation among them seems to be becoming increasingly blurred. There is a compelling need to incorporate some of the new approaches into the treatment model, to develop a greater eclecticism in therapy. For this to be done successfully, much study and research is required. Some of the aspects of therapy on the frontier are genetic counseling; sophisticated child care practices; drugs such as phenothiazine, lithium carbonate, or their derivatives; family therapy; adequate periods of controlled regression in the acute psychoses; stable working relationships with staff; and post psychotic programs of rehabilitation.

With a concerted effort, and drawing upon many perspectives and disciplines, we will undoubtedly be able to develop new models for therapy in the years ahead.

When we first opened our psychiatric unit of eleven beds at Michael Reese Hospital in 1939 (which eventually doubled to twenty-two beds), we had a wide variety of patients. They represented all ages and degreess of disturbance and a variety of diagnoses. When our new institute with eighty beds opened in 1951, the same held true, though psychosomatic and children's units had been added, both of which were eventually converted into general wards. One group of patients who early seemed to require special care and specially trained personnel were the adolescents.

In its growing superspecialization or compartmentalization, medicine had early recognized that children were not small adults, but have specific problems of their own. Even within this field, subspecialties had developed, and pediatrics was divided into work with neonates, infants, and toddlers, etc. In psychiatry, adolescence continued to attract particular attention because of the demands and pressures imposed on that stage of the life cycle by social conditions—pressures that sometimes manifest themselves in delinquency and drug abuse.

In biological research, the phrase *critical period* indicates a border or boundary through which a jump-step is made and after which change, growth, etc., are different. Learning, socialization, and acculturalization in humans are profoundly altered after critical periods have been reached. Unfortunately, not enough attention has been paid to the significance of phasic divisions in life, apart from their assignment to different specialties.

We do not know the boundaries or the timing (critical periods) of each phase and can only characterize them as phases of development, growth, maturity, decline, illness, or death. Except for the last phase, progression may be interrupted by regression to a previous temporal phase, either temporarily or permanently.

The study of each phase requires specific kinds of multidisciplinary teams; it cannot be carried out by clinical specialties alone. This means that departmental lines must be broken down as early as the first year of medical school, when each phase of the life cycle must be recognized as having its own structure-function, susceptibilities, coping mechanisms, and predominant types of breakdown.

I believe that this systematic way of relating medical sciences to the life cycle of health and disease can appropriately contribute to a logical organization of education. It is quite apparent that an understanding of the development of the human, as contrasted with the lower animals, must take into account the increasing complexities that accentuate individuality in the higher species.

Genetics or heredity, etc., is the "given" with which an organism is born, yet the genetic background cannot manifest itself except through transactions with environmental releasing mechanisms. Furthermore, genetic processes are not only apparent to some degree at birth, but may influence the entire process of development, including the character and timing of aging and death. Thus, the genetic framework maintains its influence during all of life.

Conversely, environments, which are social and cultural processes, are limiting factors. These are relatively constant, if one considers the social and cultural "surround" within a civilization, and they are part of a general process, not restricted to specific ethnic and social groups. They are part of a larger pattern of social and cultural evolution on one hand, and rapidly revolutionary changes on the other.

The recognition of the emotional and psychological constellations that are characteristic of each phase in the life cycle have led us to focus our research on specific age-groups. In turn, we have tended to organize the psychiatric hospital itself into peer groups—units that can provide viable therapy, "research opportunities," as well as social groupings that can be meaningful and supportive.

The study of human beings obviously begins with the relatively *undifferentiated infant,* who seems to be derived from a particular genetic background and is born into a particular civilization. The infant's genetic differences are only partially revealed by morphological defects. Genetic variations, such as potentialities or drive strengths, can be surmised by observing the degree of activity and the complexity of the random motor movements of the infant. *Secretory* and *endocrine differences* of genetic origin are frequently only manifested when the organism is challenged in life.

The *toddler stage* is one of considerable differentiation in which the organism has now incorporated within its psychosomatic systems memory traces derived from its experiences in its particular environment. Thus, the mother-child, father-child, child-child, child-school, child-church, and many other relationships differentiate the organism. The resulting variables, which are the subsystems of this stage, may not all be fully developed, but they are the sources of possible compensations. Thus, if a mother-child relationship is defective, a child-peer relationship may compensate for that later. Differentiation in this stage is based upon learning—and I mean not only cognitive and emotional learning, but also *physical* learning. This may involve the reinforcement of conditioned reflexes, releasing of the mechanisms of innate properties, and the imitation by incorporation of memory of images of both psychic and somatic experiences, resulting in so-called identifications (Mahler, 1971).

The third phase in the life-style of the individual is expressed in *adolescence.* It includes his somatic behaviors, personality, and coping devices, which remain relatively constant. One can surmise that new coping devices are rarely learned later in life.

The fourth stage which is appropriate to *young and middle adult life,* is characterized by varying degrees of health and varying degrees of proneness to disintegrations or disease. The proneness or susceptibility requires suitable environmental agencies for an overt state of sickness to occur. Health may persist in a relative sense until the aging process reveals the wearing out of certain tissues or systems (possibly genetically determined), in which case the system moves then to the phase of dying and death.

The fifth phase is the stage of *aging,* characterized by disease or illness related to the wearing processes. Disease is an expression of the effect of a particular environmental influence on the organism developed to this stage of life, with particular past experiences and genetic background. In chronic illness, the disease state manifests itself without much shift. The acute phase may be transient and reversible to the prone condition, but then greater degrees of reversibility are rarely possible.

In the last phase, the person has assumed a career as a patient, whose only future is in dying, a death which ultimately has an effect on others, in the mourning process (Bozzetti and MacMurray, 1977).

One can diagram this series of events in the form of a *semicircle.* Thus, the infant struggles against gravity and gradually moves upright into the erect posture of the adult. Slowly, as he grows older, he moves down again and finally gravity wins out and he is leveled to the ground. Of course, there are shortcuts to this phase of dying and death, which can occur in any period of development. The schizophrenic sometimes says that the life cycle is a journey from the womb to the tomb, and he chooses not to go through all the viscissitudes of life and makes a direct journey by suicide. If we move from this brief description of phases of development and regression to the many disciplines involved in their study, we find that they represent different methods of approach.

The need for a multidisciplinary approach to the life sciences has previously been discussed.

Supposing that, for the purpose of sound pedagogy and for a clearer understanding of process, we utilize not individual departments, such as anatomy, physiology, biochemistry, or pathology, but assign to the task multidisciplinary teams, including appropriate clinicians and social scientists.

Such a new curricular direction would be not entirely medical. Some of its aspects could be incorporated in nonmedical areas in the university, perhaps in the premedical years. At any rate, the curriculum must be conceived of as a continuous process. Its real purpose is to give to the student a concept of the totality of the life cycle, the transactional relationship among its parts, the components of the parts; to avoid reductionism on the one hand and humanism on the other. The ideal is to present a full picture and then fill in the details, not only with contributions from scientific disciplines, but also with insights drawn from the specialties of the applied medical sciences. Though it would then be necessary to sift through a variety of approaches and differences of methods, the total picture could give meaning to a total life concept containing both so-called healthy and sick components. This is an example of unitary thinking.

Within the medical specialties as they are compartmentalized in departments, there are "core areas" that must be taught and within which experience by practice is necessary for adequate mastery, by all physicians, no matter where their professional paths will take them.

There is another core area basic to the education of all graduate students, no matter what their specialty or apparent career goals. This is a knowledge of the *health-illness* system—a system that cannot be fractured, since it denotes a process in continuity throughout the life span.

Each phase in the life cycle has its characteristic internal processes, its specific stresses and capacities for defense, coping, and reconstitution. Each and the whole have their interfaces with specific sociocultural environments, their ecosystems. As I have stressed many times, such understanding of the total life cycle transcends departmental lines; it combines knowledge of laboratory procedures, life in pairs, families, groups, and the larger society. It is concerned with phases of stability, stress responses, and repair.

A curriculum based on these concepts would give the student a broad biopsychosocial education as an adequate theoretical framework within which overall understanding of life, illness, and dying may be achieved. Once having grasped the principles and details of specific subsystems, fields, or specialties through such a multidisciplinary approach, the student is then ready to enrich his knowledge through learning and experience. The fractionated concepts of organisms will then have been put together. Once the field, system, and transactional processes become understood and used, they will spread out into ever-widening fields of thought.

As we know, the current trend is toward a division of the total life cycle into phases with specific characteristics, both of maturation and decline, development, and regression with physiological, psychological, and behavioral expressions. Psychoanalytic theory has further divided the life cycle into ever finer phases based on dominant ways of thinking, feeling, and behaving, corresponding to the maturation of physical zones, such as oral, anal, phallic, and genital, and those phases have been subdivided again according to vectors of incorporation, retention, and expulsion. The discipline now called *child development* has also recognized even finer phases within childhood related to cognitive and conative complexities.

The criteria for differentiation are difficult to set if we use chronological age alone. We have loosely attempted to resolve this difficulty by adding the words *early* or *late,* but such designations are still more or less arbitrary. Late adolescence, for instance, may be a phase really belonging to young adulthood. If the phasic differentiation of the life cycle requires differential diagnostic and therapeutic approaches, then we should learn the state and trait characteristics and the several socioeconomic-cultural environments impinging on them.

Unfortunately, psychiatrists have based their approach on experiences with the pathological from which they extrapolate to what they define as healthy or normal for a particular phase. As a result, we are caught in a mesh of myths, such as the idea that adolescents must go through a period of turbulence in order to become healthy adults. My own research on homoclites, who resolved their problems by action, introspected little, and, as "muscular Christians," had little ambition to make money but wanted to help other people, were considered "sick" by my critics. This group has been described in detail in Chapter 8.

I believe that the serious student of adolescence must be cautious in using the parameter of age and should skeptically question a sharp health illness dichotomy. At every age, maturation and development are accompanied by regression and decline, the algebraic sum of which varies within a wide range constituting the many varieties of normality or health.

For the past five years, Offer, Mahron, and Ostrov (In press) of Michael Reese Hospital have studied juvenile delinquents, admitted to Illinois State Psychiatric Institute, who had performed serious antisocial acts and were in need of psychiatric treatment. None were schizophrenic or mentally retarded. Half were male and half female. Two-thirds were white and one-third black. Each patient was in the hospital for a minimum of three months. Psychiatric treatment was given to individuals as indicated.

The subjects were studied via a host of behavioral, psychological, psychiatric-biological, and sociopsychological instruments. All parents were studied, as well as the staff on the units. The variables were correlated and factor and cluster analyzed through a method similar to that used in the Normal Adolescent Study.

Four statistically valid and clinically meaningful psychodynamic subgroups of delinquent adolescents were found. These were derived from the ongoing treatment program and investigative research project. The genesis of psychodynamic thinking about delinquency, its causes and its treatment, leads to the exposition of the four subgroups: the impulsive, the narcissistic, the depressed, and the borderline.

The *impulsive delinquent* shows more violent and nonviolent antisocial behavior. He is considered quite disturbed by his therapist, socially insensitive by his teachers, and unlikeable and quick to action by most staff members. Yet, he seems to have some awareness of a need for help. His delinquency derives from a propensity for action and immediate discharge of tension.

The *narcissistic delinquent* sees himself as well adjusted and not delinquent. However, parents and staff recognize his difficulties in adapting and characterize him as resistant, cunning, manipulative, and superficial. He denies problems, only *appears* to engage in therapy, exaggerates his own self-worth, and in his delinquency tends to use others for his own needs, especially to help regulate his self-esteem.

The *depressed delinquent* shows school initiative, is liked by staff, and tries to engage with staff therapeutically. Relationships with parents lead to strongly internalized value systems, and these delinquents tend to show structuralized or neurotic conflicts, from which delinquent behavior serves as a relief.

The *borderline delinquent* is a passive, emotionally empty, and depleted person, who is not well liked, is an outcast sometimes, needy and clinging at other times, and whose future seems pessimistic. These adolescents behave delinquently to prevent psychotic disintegration or fusion and to relieve themselves of internal desolation.

The subgroups are found in all of the demographic cells studied and contribute to our understanding of adolescent delinquent behavior, regardless of age, sex, socioeconomic status, or color. The results are expressed in forms of feeling, thinking, and behavior more or less organized into an adaptive whole suitable for coping or not coping with the exigencies of life. The end results depend upon the repertoire of internalized social roles and the maintenance of a healthy balance by defenses against overwhelming stresses, or the capacity for restitution when such defenses are temporarily overcome. In fact, we as psychiatrists frequently underevaluate the capacities of humans to defend, compensate, and restitute in the face of the unexpectable environmental changes.

Currently, we are experiencing a shift from materialistic to moralistic values, which is creating a precarious balance at all ages, particularly adolescence. In the United States, a group has "dropped out" of the mainstream of the life of technology into a drug society, which frequently results in irreparable damage. Another group fights against our current establishment, hoping to change it prior to their necessary and ultimate commitment. Another group completely avoids affectionate involvement with any other human being and ends with the stable instability of the borderline.

Whether biological, psychological, or social systems are studied, there is a teleological necessity for supraordinate and organized function of control and regulation. As psychiatrists, we know how differentiation of part-functions and hence interacting part-objects are integrated by a supraordinate ego as only one example of natural processes at all levels. To generalize, living systems at all levels are characterized by a principle of order that stabilizes and preserves a total pattern composed of semiautonomous parts.

Nevertheless, there is more to life than stability and regulation of order for which external favorable environments, situations, and goals are sought to maintain physio– and psychological homeostasis. Although change arouses considerable anxiety in individuals, families, and groups, there is a progressive trend toward goal-changing behaviors. These are basic to what are called *evolution, individual growth, development,* and *creativity.* Each creates a positive feedback reinforcing changes in thinking and behavior and progressing toward our hypothetical humanism.

Thus, instead of referring to dichotomies and conflict, we may refer to two processes inextricably linked: Stability and change. L.L. Whyte's (1948) phrase sums this up: "Unity in diversity and continuity in change," or unified thinking characteristic of a systems approach. This is contrasted with dualistic thinking oriented only toward stability and permanence based on the illusion generated by objective science that some parts or variables and especially our terrestial background can be viewed as steady.

Unitary thinking, on the other hand, considers that both parts and whole, both focus and background, are constantly changing, but regulated by some form of organization that prevents dedifferentiation, focal cancerous overgrowth, internal psychological confusion, social chaos, and anarchy. Our problem is to identify the ways by which the organizational principle operates.

We have seen that, during the years sixteen to nineteen, the adolescent completes many aspects of mature development and is still working on others. By age nineteen, young people are physically mature and are most likely to have attained their peak cognitive development, though knowledge can continuously increase. Psychosocial development, on the other hand, has come a long way but is by no means complete (Peterson, in press). Forming an identity is the major psychosocial task of adolescence, but the development of some aspects of identity continues throughout life for many of us. Some aspects of psychosocial development also appear to be dependent upon cognitive development and therefore may be limited by it.

The development of identity at age nineteen using Erikson's

framework, is summarized: Most youth of this age have achieved temporal perspective and, in fact, appear to have a heightened awareness of time. Self-certainty is a more difficult task to master, and many individuals continue some degree of self-consciousness throughout life. Egocentrism is less prevalent by age nineteen.

Many youths nineteen years of age are still actively experimenting with roles. For others, role fixation is a realistic limitation on future opportunities. By age nineteen, most youths are beginning, at least, to consider occupational choices. Most have begun to develop intimate relationships.

The last two conflicts of the adolescent crisis—leader– and fellowship versus authority confusion, and ideological commitment versus confusion of values—are less likely to be resolved by age nineteen. Most college-aged youths are actively struggling with these issues, and relatively few have actually resolved them much before the end of college.

The Offers' study demonstrates that about one-fourth of their modal sample progressed continuously and developed values similar to those of their parents. A second group developed by spurts with periodic turmoil. The third group experienced the years from fourteen to twenty-two with the turmoil frequently generalized to all adolescents. For them, the developmental tasks leading to an identity were difficult.

There is good evidence that parents are especially important to adolescent development. Well-adjusted parents can facilitate development in this period, while conflicted parents may exacerbate difficulties.

Although the field of child development has become extremely active in response to the information vacuum indicated above, progress has been made mostly in the understanding of somatic rather than psychological development. The striking exception is the work of Anna Freud (1957) and her colleagues, which extends over three decades. Her monograph summarizes this extensive research and is a beacon for current and future progress in the study of child development in health and illness. She indicates the powerful influence of the environment on the child, in contrast to many analysts concerned exclusively with internal innate forces. Yet, external factors alone are not pathogenic agents. In this statement, we see that the continuum-concept in etiology has finally been accepted. Experience is interpreted by the growing organism according to the phase-adequate complexes, affects, anxieties, and fantasies that are aroused by them. The child's position in a curve of psychological growth is a function of maturation, adaptation, and structuralization. The child's needs require an environment that can satisfy them. In fact, the child has to teach its mother how to mother him so that he may learn to differentiate from her. Anna Freud points out the error of the concept of steadily progressive maturation and adaptation. Psychological development is associated with unequal shifts and periods of regression. "Constant forward and backward movements, progression and regression, alternate and interact with each other." She stresses the difficulty in determining criteria of health and illness and the inadequacy of our diagnostic classifications, as well as our prognostic indices.

It is impossible to enumerate the evidences of progress in theory and practice developed by Anna Freud's group. Briefly, it has looked clearly at the processes of psychological growth, using the observational techniques of general psychiatry, the psychoanalytic techniques of child analysis, both verbal and play, and the observational techniques of the child development field. For example (A. Freud, 1957), "Obviously, what determines the direction of development are not the major infantile events and constellations in themselves but a multitude of accompanying circumstances, the consequences of which are difficult to judge both retrospectively in adult analysis and prognostically in the assessment of children." Based on these concepts, Anna Freud and her co-workers have established a useful index derived from process studies from which great advances in our knowledge of health and illness should accrue. Even more important for the progress of psychoanalysis than the broad statements made by Anna Freud of the "openness" and multifactorial processes in growth and development in health and illness and in therapeutic success and failure are her sharp and clear statements. All of these are so clearly defined that they may be considered as hypotheses essential for the testing of psychoanalytic theory by a variety of methods.

Progress in the field of child psychiatry has been regrettably slow. When our new institute opened in 1951, it was served by a part-time child psychiatrist and a skilled child psychiatric nurse. Unfortunately, there were few well-trained and experienced child psychiatrists available for this unit of twelve beds, which contained badly disturbed children who exhibited violent behavior.

Alexander greatly damaged the field of child psychiatry in the 1930s, and it still suffers from its early neglect. Despite the fact that several of the Chicago group intensively studied child psychiatry and child analysis with Anna Freud (Margaret Gerard, Helen Ross, and George Mohr), they were given little opportunity for further development. Alexander stubbornly believed that the problems of children were all due to their parents. It was not necessary to treat the child; what was important was to treat only the mother, father, or both. All three of the above analysts left the field—at least for a long time—and only later, after Alexander left Chicago, were child analysis, child psychiatry, and child care supported, but it will be many decades before Chicago can make up the time lost. In Chicago, child psychiatrists are a scarce species, and they have isolated themselves from the mainstream.

At P & PI the cost of our unit was too great and the results too poor to justify continuation. We had to close it, and the repercussions were the most damaging of my administration. Our decision, which was in truth solely an administrative one, was considered "antichild." The Pritzker Children's Center, an active residential treatment center for children staffed by graduate students, had been established at the nearby University of Chicago. Its major difficulty had continued to be its lack of endowment and its year-to-year deficit, which was largely a result of its original attempt to imitate the heavily endowed Orthogenic School of Bruno Bettleheim, which could support children for seven to ten years, far into adolescence.

In the face of constant administrative and economic difficulties, I received almost yearly appeals for our Institute to take over the management of Pritzker. After its first director became ill and resigned, we participated in a holding operation for one year while a new director was being recruited. Dr. Jean Spurlock carried on the professional activities with great efficiency. With the advent of a new director, there was a gradual turn around of professional programs, and income from short-term patients, third-party payers, and state and local communities eventually turned deficit into solvency.

The Jewish Federation and its agencies have tended for a long time to shift funds away from hospital support to social agencies. Such an effort is, in my opinion, misguided. The Jewish Children's Bureau, which had the responsibility for the Pritzker Center, eventually wanted to divest itself of the responsibility and again approached us. Now that Pritzker was solvent, we were more receptive, and a merger was accomplished, despite the continuous struggle with the University of Chicago.

It clearly made sense for Pritzker and Reese's P & PI to merge, so that each could profit by the experiences and expertise of the other in the development of continuity of the rehabilitation processes. Therefore, the Pritzker Children's Center became a section of the Reese Department of Psychiatry while maintaining its professional autonomy and sense of direction, assisted by the research capabilities of the Reese Psychiatric Institute. Prevention, diagnosis, and rehabilitation of psychologically disturbed children should improve as a result of this merger.

The young adult group in the hospital soon came to demand separate consideration as they observed the extra consideration given to the adolescents, and they too were constituted as a peer group. Special personnel developed experience in treating these young adults whose major life problem was choice of careers and maintenance of jobs. We employed a job counselor who helped a great deal. This peer group also contained a large number of acute schizophrenics, young depressives, and borderline patients who served as valuable research material.

The fourth group was not segregated with special services, because they were middle-aged patients, the traditional objects of rehabilitation by psychotherapy, psychopharmacology, and sometimes electroshock treatment.

The final peer group established at P & PI under the leadership of Finkel included the aged, who only recently have aroused the interest of psychiatrists. Previously dismissed as having cerebral arteriosclerosis or senile brain changes, they were usually afforded little study and little or no treatment. One of my residents startled me one day by asserting that an elderly patient of his had no psychodynamics!

It is generally believed that early life patterns are intensified in old age, and that whatever hope is generated is based on past patterns of optimism. But all old people have problems (otherwise there would be no life), and they resolve them through inertia, depression, obsessions, and paranoia, etc. For many, there is extreme fear of poverty; many assert unreasonable independence; and some irrationally state that time seems to jump too fast. It is interesting that many older people are kept out of hospitals by older internists, who give up their own hospital practices except for emergencies, to make frequent house calls day or night.

Although our staff and those at other institutions have worked long and hard to establish peer groups, perfect their management, and follow them into home, school, jobs, outpatient facilities, halfway houses, and final disposition, little information is available about any of these facets of peer group treatment. My own task as an administrator has been to facilitate space, staff, and salaries for the peer groups, but I have not participated personally in any. From a distance, the patients who were members of all groups seemed to profit from their treatment, but little has been written or spoken about therapy and practically nothing about results except a monograph by Garber (1972), who followed up our adolescent patients for ten years. From previous experience, I suspect that all groups except the young adults and the middle-aged adults continue their position as "high risks" all their lives. The geriatric patients die in greater emotional stability, the young adults develop their share of schizophrenia, and the middle adults are reasonably well rehabilitated. But the children before puberty continue to be sick, and the adolescents have a questionable future.

The peer groups in our hospital were, in fact, little more than specialized therapeutic groups about whom the staff learned a great deal. Little research has been developed from these services.

Historically, the adolescent group originated in 1953; the young adult group began shortly thereafter. The middle adult group was composed of the traditional rehabilitating persons requiring milieu therapy, psychotherapy, and medication. The geriatric group consisted of men and women from age sixty-two years and up. The staff for all of these groups comprised a psychiatrist, psychologist, resident, an actitvity leader, social worker, and recreation leader. With no systemic research, all I can state is that the patients felt better and behaved more normally as they associated socially with their contemporaries.

CHAPTER 13

Psychoanalysis

NO ONE WHO HAS TAKEN THE TIME to become familiar with the theory and practice of psychoanalysis would deny the seminal influence of this field on psychiatry and the broader social sciences. Although it started as a movement, and although the early meetings of a few psychoanalysts with Freud, each wearing an identifying ring, seem like the religious conclaves of cardinals, as younger psychiatrists have joined the ranks, their solidarity has weakened. In fact, in the United States, many local societies under the domination of the American Psychoanalytic Association split in two because of conflicts and personal antagonisms. There has been an effort, however, to preserve the strong "center core." Criticisms from without have been considered to be based on ignorance or resistance. Those from within have been ascribed to analytic failures, but if one looks at the large number of so-called mature teaching analysts who are faithful members of the Establishment, it is evident that their personal psychoanalysis has done less for them than they expect from their students.

Thousands of articles and books have been written about psychoanalysis and about Freud—praising, criticizing, and distorting his work. It must be remembered that the standard against which the field is viewed is based on its own self-image as "our science." It is considered by the faithful to be not merely a humanistic or existential field, but a naturalistic science open to criticism and revision. Yet, paradoxically, any statement depreciating or challenging any aspect of the field or its founder is open to inaccurate and undocumented attack.

My own critiques of psychoanalysis—never directed against Freud himself—have been published in Marmor's *Modern Psycho-*

analysis (1968) and in my book, *Psychiatry in Broad Perspective* (1975d). Freud knew that the major critiques would come from America, and we have already discussed the reasons for his personal biases against the New World. Although Ernest Jones (1955) made an earnest attempt to portray Freud's life impartially in his three-volume biography, he in fact hurt Freud's image by distorted history with poor insight. To dwell on other attacks and misinterpretations, justified or not, would be fruitless. And what is more, the angry responses to criticism have done no credit to the analytic profession. One such response should be singled out for mention, however—that of Gitelson (Grinker, 1965b)—which was an unnecessary and ill-advised overreaction.

Despite claims to the contrary, psychoanalysis does not possess the rigor of a true science. Bronowski (1977) does not accept the excuse that exact predictions cannot yet be made because of the immaturity of the field of psychology. Psychologies are limited severely and constantly by the self-references underlying them. Bronowski quotes Popper (1959) to the effect that psychoanalysis, derived from the unconscious, which he calls Freud's "invention," is especially filled with the paradoxes produced by self-references.

I have traced the evolution of the field from its beginnings through the adoption of structural theory and the abandonment of psychoanalytic metapsychology, libido, and psychic energy, to its confluence with general systems theory. I presented this historical analysis in modified form as the fourteenth Karen Horney Lecture (1966a). Merton Gill and Philip Holzman (1976) have put their own stamp on the discussion by stating categorically that "there is therefore no direct connection between metapsychology and psychology." In fact, they see metapsychology as a natural science framework of force, energy, and structure, while psychological propositions deal with intention and meaning. What this amounts to, unfortunately, is a mind-body dichotomy. How are they to be brought together? What constitutes a unified theory?

Psychoanalysis has developed concepts that can be defined as holistic as far as they are concerned with intra-psychic processes. Psychoanalytic "metapsychology" is a system of high-level abstraction serving as an umbrella for the structural, economic, dynamic, and adaptational theories, few of which are defined sufficiently enough that testable hypotheses may be derived from them. Yet, leading psychoanalytic theorists consider that their metapsychology is also a general theory of psychology. Freud's metapsychology (his "witch," as he calls it) is by far the most encompassing (and satisfying) theoretical framework on which to place an intrapsychic phenomenon. But it can only be a part of a general systems theory, since it is unidisciplinary and cannot be extrapolated to biological, ecological, and social sciences—no matter how often its adherents state that it can explain all of human behavior.

The basic "mythology" (Freud's own word) of psychoanalysis is its instinct theory, which postulates that libido with its pressures or energies, sometimes called *psychic energy,* arises from various somatic foci and endures vicissitudes in which personality, character, health, or illness are determined. This hydraulic model had powerful heuristic value in the early part of the twentieth century and therefore only reluctantly is it abandoned today, when current opinion indicates that it is information and not energy that is the measure of brain activity. As Marcus (1962) points out, chromosomes define only the direction of development; learning and experience furnish precise details. Likewise, instinctual processes are the manifestation of a complex control and communication system, and libido is not some metaphysical chemical system diffusing a fluidlike psychic energy.

Concepts of psychological energy, libido, and specific drives are now being gradually replaced by modern information theory. Man is seen as involved in various quantities of information exchanges—too little, too much, or incompatible exchange. Such qualities and quantities of information act upon all levels of the organism at all times. One important current task is to investigate the qualities of communication between the child and his human environment, which determines specific patterns of personality, character, and proneness to serious stress responses.

There is also an ongoing debate as to what psychoanalysis is supposed to do. We have heard a great deal about encouraging insight, but this is a wobbly definition. Perhaps the patient learns to accept his limitations, or to be able to love, work, play, and be optimistic, or to weaken the severity of the superego. Probably change within the patient occurs after he successfully attempts new forms of action. Perhaps this in itself is insight.

In 1911, Ernest Jones presented a paper before the Chicago Neurological Society. He split the speciality into two camps; those violently opposed and those eager to learn and understand the "new psychology" (Grinker, 1963a). The senior neurologist, Hugh T. Patrick, gave serious and understanding consideration to psychonanalysis. Julius Grinker stated:

> It must be admitted that it is not very easy to understand Freud's viewpoint, and for that reason we are under obligation to the essayist [Jones] who has in numerous contributions and discussions endeavored to acquaint the American profession with Freud's work. The physician who does not practice psychoanalysis in the broader sense is not competent to treat nervous cases. The man who either had no experience with the method or else is too indolent to learn it, is a very poor critic indeed and had better learn something about it.
>
> This new psychotherapy has as its basis a plausible psychology, splendid reasoning, and a profound acquaintance with the innermost depth of human nature. Regardless of whether Freud's psycho-analytic method will ever become popular in therapeutics, it has certainly opened our eyes to facts hitherto completely ignored or not at all recognized.

My father, blinded by his later sad misinterpretation of transferences, denounced the field and refused to support my efforts to become analyzed and to learn about it. My own psychoanalytic training and analysis by Freud after my father's death were discussed previously.

Many others took a harshly critical view of the Jones paper, as well, and denounced psychoanalytic theory or methods. But the controversy did not last long, because those who tried the method were soon overwhelmed by transference reactions of love and hate from their patients. Only one psychiatrist persisted, talking but writing little. Indeed, Dr. Ralph Hamill was the only Chicago psychiatrist who became a charter member of the American Psychoanalytic Association, along with Dr. James J. Putnam of Boston, president; Ernest Jones of Toronto, secretary; Trigant Burrow, John T. MacCurdy, Adolf Meyer, and G. Lane Taneyhill of Baltimore; and G. Alexander Young of Omaha.

Ilse Bry (1962) has written of these early days in a personal communication: "The well-known period of articulate opposition to psychoanalysis had been preceded by a period of equally articulate appreciation which was later obscured and forgotten. It is intriguing to note how often the same individuals who had first made a sincere effort to assimilate Freud's ideas later changed their mind and their attitude."

Bry and Rifkin (1964) would like to draw a line of thinking of scientific consistency rather than historical continuity through the half-century from 1911 to 1961. There is a nucleus of truth in this idea. Currently, there is within the psychoanalytic profession a growing criticism of theory and methods not based on prudery, ignorance, or emotionality, but on a sophisticated attitude by persons whose training is more scientific. These people's vistas have also become wider, because they have had more contact with other fields than did the earlier members of the profession, who were more completely immersed in the psychoanalytic discipline.

The story of psychoanalysis in America has been told by several others, but I would like to add a subjective account of what I have observed on the Chicago scene. After the first fiasco at the University of Chicago, Alexander moved to Boston, where he studied criminals with a lawyer named Hugo Staub. As I have mentioned, he returned to Chicago in 1932 to found a new psychoanalytic institute, with a mixed faculty of experienced analysts from Europe and a group of young, freshly trained students.

The one departure from Chicago that created a stir was that of Karen Horney, who not only moved to New York, but who also established an independent institute and society, significantly emphasizing social and cultural factors, in contrast to the biological (instinct theories of Freud) in the etiology and treatment of the neuroses. Freud was not surprised at this move, stating that Alexander had known Horney in Berlin and never should have taken her to Chicago! Surprisingly, I was invited by the Association for the Advancement of Psychoanalysis, although I was not a member, to give the Fourteenth Annual Karen Horney Lecture, entitled "Open-Systems' Psychiatry." Horney certainly emphasized what had been excluded from psychoanalysis in its closed-system period. Neurotic conflicts were considered by her as more than internal drive derivatives. I pointed out that, in this era of open systems, we no longer need splinter groups emphasizing this or that. But splinter groups develop lives of their own and persist long after their usefulness is over.

The Chicago Institute for Psychoanalysis was under Alexander's direction from its founding in 1932 until 1956. Its relations with the local society and the national organization are described, and then how it has functioned in the care of patients, education, and research is discussed.

It is clear that the society was organized by a handful of people before the analytic institute existed and was not involved in training. Alexander wanted the new institute to be an academic organization independent from the society with a faculty responsible for training. Members of the society who were not on the faculty were welcome to attend conferences and seminars. The society did not control the institute as in other cities, but in an indirect way, served as a postgraduate forum. Later the society "screened" graduates from the institute for membership, but I do not know of many who were turned down.

The main goal for the new institute was to establish a free and liberal organization with new ideas open to all analysts. Alexander had broad interests and sought out and participated in local academic, medical, and psychiatric activities. As more students were graduated, some indoctrinated by an antagonistic group, more resistance against new approaches developed, and conflict within the organization increased. In those early years, the various North American local societies were banded together into a federation. As time went on, the conservative, and often reactionary, group in the country turned the national organization into an overall association with each society an affiliate subject to the same general rules and regulations.

As a result, general rules, regulations, and procedures, which all component institutes and societies were expected to follow, were laid down by the American Federation. Accreditation of new local organizations, disaccreditations, surveys, and number of hours were rigidly controlled. Graduation from a local institute did not mean easy access to the American. This was only possible through lengthy documentation of patients analyzed and extensive paperwork that discouraged many from applying.

Alexander fought vigorously against the requirement of four-day-a-week analyses and other dictatorial directives from the American Federation, but he lost. On the other hand, the Establishment wanted to require its own students to be certified by the diplomate board of the American Federation alone. The Academy of Psychoanalysis objected to this inbred control—and won.

In the meantime, the younger analysts in Chicago objected to the procedures for obtaining membership in the American Association, and many never applied. Conversely, the newly educated analysts of Alexander's day became progressively more compliant and orthodox. In fact, Alexander's early retirement and departure from Chicago for Los Angeles was at least partially due to his staff's discontent and their open revolt against his liberality. Among these liberal attitudes was his three-day-a-week analyses, his "betrayal" of the libido theory, his manipulation of the transference by "role playing," and finally his attempt to move the Chicago Institute out from control of the American Establishment.

Benedek (1956) has contrasted the free and open communications among the faculty when the institute was small with today's controlled competitive fears and jealousies within a large group of three analytic generations. There is currently little unity of purpose. With the present generation, psychoanalysis is not the center of their professional life. Only about 20 percent of their patients are in analysis. They are engaged in many other ventures and projects that are much more eclectic than those of their psychoanalytic ancestors.

The use of the term *training* by psychoanalytic institutes (as opposed to *education*) early set the climate for a technological approach rather than a graduate education in an academic environment. Alexander realized this, but he could do nothing to change the emphasis except to pursue his desire to be an academician. Thus, he joined my clinical conferences at the University of Chicago and later became a faculty member of the University of Illinois Medical College from 1938 to 1956. His pleas for the development of psychoanalytic departments within universities were futile.

Philip Holzman (1973) has addressed the question of the most appropriate setting for the psychoanalytic institute of the future and has pleaded for an adjustment in the course and direction that psychoanalytic education has taken:

> If the function of psychoanalytic training institutes is to train practitioners of psychoanalytic technique, it is unreasonable to expect institutes to offer effective training in research or other scholarly applications of psychoanalysis. But if one insists that the training of psychoanalysts should, at least in some instances, encompass more than the teaching of psychoanalytic therapy, the training institutes have been failing in their function to educate candidates for scholarly activities. Whether the structure of the independent training institutes can permit such broadened training is questioned. One solution is to move the educational function into the university setting.

Since I was part of the institute's early training programs, I can describe them firsthand. I had set up a small psychiatric unit at Billings Hospital, to the dismay of the professor of surgery. Alexander and Leon Saul helped me start weekly inpatient conferences, Jules Masserman (rescued from a state hospital in Maryland) was my first psychiatric resident, and Helen Richter Gilmore, now at Yale, was my first psychiatric intern. I immediately entered the training program at the Chicago Institute despite only one year of personal analysis with Freud.

The general attitude of the faculty at that time was that the students were adults able to learn through experience and their own selected readings. There was no prescription for the number of so-called control patients (supervision), no set number of hours and no specified time spread for supervision. One of my supervisors told me to return whenever I needed to, but I cherished Dr. French's careful and profound help and understanding.

I must say that our choice of patients for analysis was not intelligent, and we often failed in our attempts to hold them in treatment. Transference interpretations were most difficult for the novice, and little help was available.

Among the students were many so-called geographic trainees, who came from Topeka, Cincinnati, and St. Louis, etc., for weekend analyses, conferences, and supervision. This weekend form of teaching was necessary because candidates had to make a living in practice or in other jobs, but it was often an obstacle to a sound psychoanalytic education. The outline of the curriculum was simple. Saturday morning was devoted to a clinical conference attended by the young faculty and students. At noon, lunch was served from the institute's kitchen, after which a book or a series of articles was reviewed, with a student leading off the discussion that followed. In the afternoon, the society (which was made up of the same people, with one or two additions) held a meeting at which a faculty member would give a paper, which would in turn be discussed by faculty and students.

Whenever a student felt that he was ready for a final examination, he would so indicate. The examination itself was brief and entirely oral, because what he knew and could do was already well recognized by the faculty. I remember that when my turn came I was ushered into a conference room and asked one question: "What is the superego?" In five minutes I was through and had received my certificate, which entitled me to become not only a member of the Chicago Society, but also of the American. Thus, there were no complicated reports of cases analyzed or a host of other ploys such as those that keep the student of today fearful, dependent, and conforming to the will of the Establishment. Nevertheless, as my friend the late M.R. Kaufman of New York, reminded me, it took at least five years of experience to really become an analyst. Dedicated, optimistic, and hard working, we studied, talked with our peers, and acquired the necessary experience.

All was not that simple for long, however, because analytic groups became more rooted in ritual, more controlling and more infantile in their conflicts. There was conflict between local institutes and societies and within institutes between liberals and conservatives (some were really orthodox). Students were treated like children. Classes were formalized, and the curriculum was planned for at least five years. Soon Alexander's liberalism was lost, and at least temporarily, the free Chicago Institute became fettered by the American Society's restrictions.

If students asked questions that were searching, skeptical, and indicated doubts, they were threatened with probation and return to more analysis, thereby stifling free discussion. Analysis of students was handicapped by the role of their analysts in supporting or denying their admission to the training program. Teaching from Freud's papers and books, even in the earliest days, were presented as historical data, without enabling the student to know what was currently acceptable.

What bothered many of us were the frequent *interminable analyses* conducted by our colleagues. When analytic theory moved from the Oedipus complex as the most important focus for change to a study of pregenital experiences and conflicts, analysts attempted to reconstruct these early experiences in the transference. Year after year was vainly wasted in an attempt to reorganize the total character structures of patients. These attempts were unrealized therapeutic ambitions, as one could observe by the wide variety of neuroses and personality and character disorders of analytic graduates.

That there is no simple correlation between therapeutic results and the length and intensity of treatment has been recognized, tacitly or explicitly, by most experienced psychoanalysts and is an old source of dissatisfaction among them.

The deeper structures of the mind, which are evolutionarily developed and characteristically programmed, are overlaid by experiences that together produce a phenotype that cannot be fragmented and united anew in a less neurotic way. The same applies to structural linguistics, which are programmed but modified by learning. As Stent (1975) states

> The great strength of Freudian analytical psychology is that it does offer a theoretical approach to understanding human behavior. Its great weakness, however, is that it is not possible to verify its propositions. And this can be said also of most other structuralist schools active in the human sciences. They do try to explain human behavior within a general theoretical framework, in contrast to their positivist

> counterparts who cannot, or rather refuse to try to do so. But there is no way of verifying the structuralist theories in the manner in which the theories of physics can be verified through critical experiments or observations. The structuralist theories are, and may forever remain, merely plausible, being, maybe, the best we can do to account for the complex phenomenon of man.

When Alexander (1961) conceived the idea that briefness in therapy should be emphasized, he began a series of investigations with other members of his staff. Unfortunately, he called this *brief psychoanalysis,* which brought down on him the wrath of most analysts in the country, except for a few of his colleagues. Brief psychotherapy would have been accepted, but not brief analysis! But the term persisted, and like the typical American bandwagon, many younger analysts hopped on but gradually dropped out. Now, the term *brief* is applied only to psychotherapy.

In the late 1940s and during the decade of the 1950s, psychoanalysis became fashionable for discontented wealthy people, mostly women, who experienced anxieties or depressions with which their culture could not cope. They sought analysts in droves. Unfortunately, some analysts avoided analyzing anger within the transference, maintaining their patients in an enthralled state of dependency for years. When their analysts died or left Chicago, the released rage within their social groups was something to behold.

Gradually, many lay people in Chicago have become disenchanted with psychoanalysis as a form of treatment. Its therapeutic results were not great, and the cost in time, energy, and money was excessive. As a result, many analysts did more psychotherapy than analysis, except for the training analysts, who seemed impervious to the realities around them. Even today, highly competent and experienced analysts put their names on lists indicating that they have free analytic hours.

Although the national survey of psychoanalytic education prepared by Lewin and Ross in 1960 included data from Chicago, it is evident that surveys of psychoanalytic education have the tendency to reveal what people say they do or what they think they do, but do not reveal what actually is done or the meaningful impact of what is accomplished, regardless of what the intent may be. Such surveys tap conscious attitudes, as contrasted with pre- or unconscious meaningful trends. In a sense, surveys always reveal the more liberal and the more avowed experimental purposes, while concealing the rigidities and the parochial. To quote from my own appraisal: "One could take all the surveys, all the righteous and well-meaning statements, and all the expressions of liberality at face value. But the real and crucial considerations of what is accomplished in education can be achieved only by examining its products. It requires not much in the way of planned examination to indicate to us in this, the deccade of the sixties, that psychoanalytic education has not been especially helpful for the advancement of psychoanalytic theory, research, or practice."

Gradually, after the loose association of psychoanalytic societies and institutes were merged into a supraordinate organization called the *American Psychoanalytic Association,* this elite controlling establishment moved free, tolerant, and open societies into a closed system, against the vigorous protests of many. The number of hours per week for psychoanalysis, the kinds of patients treated, the appointment of training analysts and supervisors, and the control of teaching methods and teachers were rigidly ruled. A Chicago subgroup promulgating a personal orthodoxy dominated our local scene. Lay analysts were forbidden, except for a favored few appointed by the New England Society.

Whatever opposition raised its head was promptly squelched, and many liberal psychoanalysts talked about splitting from the American Association, raising the anxiety titer in many of us. Alexander, defeated by the institute he had founded and developed, left Chicago before his retirement age for Los Angeles for a new career.

Alexander (1966) closed his last work on psychoanalysis with a passage that amply describes his progressive leadership:

> Just because so much still has to be explored, we must not only tolerate but encourage individual differences, personal initiative of teachers and also of the students, instead of insisting on strict uniformity and conformity. We must return to local autonomy of institutes from a uniformly systematized centrally regulated educational

> system. In view of the great many existing uncertainties in the theory of treatment, we are far from being ripe for the degree of standardization we adopted some years ago. If we continue with the present educational policies, the best qualified group, the psychoanalysts, will lose leadership in developing Freud's heritage. Then not we but the rapidly growing borderline group of psychoanalytically oriented psychiatrists who are unhampered by rules and the dogmatic censorship of their conferes will accomplish the inevitable reforms necessary for training effective practitioners.

"Psychiatry is not a science, psychoanalysis is a basic science of individual psychology." These are apparently strong phrases used by Gitelson (1965), denying the scientific basis of psychiatry and allocating to psychoanalysis the position of being basic, but they give the lie to meaningful language. There is a turnabout nature to this declaration since for decades the criticism has been leveled that psychoanalysis is not a science.

In the late 1960s and early 1970s, the students of the local institutes revolted against the oppressive tactics of their faculties. The criteria for admission to training and the maintenance within the educational pathway became less strict. Training of nonmedical persons for research and even therapy became widespread. Programs under the auspices of the American Association for the Advancement of Science (AAAS) were started by the Academy. In general, we can state that the closed system gradually opened. Psychologists, social workers, and teachers were trained at the psychoanalytic institutes. Anthropologists and social scientists were included in the faculties. A variety of journals not belonging to the American Association began to thrive. Slowly the openness of the pre-American days, closed by the American's control, has now returned.

This is fine, but subsequent to Freud, all psychoanalysts who could write attempted to verify, modify, or deny parts of Freud's theories. This they called *research*. For the most part, the results have been pitiful. Papers read at meetings and published today sound like those we heard and read twenty to forty years ago. Where are the hard data? They are not present, except for an occasional abstract. What is the full extent of the dyadic communication system? Why do we hear about metapsychology instead of empirical data with explicit statements of numbers of patients, reliability, and validation written in understandable language instead of jargon composed of words with multiple meanings?

Just recently a panel report from the National Conference on Psychoanalytic Education and Research was published by the American Psychoanalytic Association. Many of the conclusions are of value, although their implementation would indeed be difficult because of student indifference and absence of scholarly atmosphere in the Institute. Without clinical psychoanalysts with research attitudes and potential as important new role models, psychoanalysis may not survive. Instead of constructive disagreement there has, up to now been destructive splitting and isolation from scientific communities in association with universities. Wisdom suggestts an institutionalization of controversy. Wallerstein (1966) emphasizes that psychoanalysis *should be* an integral part of the wider intellectual academic world, what I have long urged, as a part of systems approach. The lack of research and scholarship applies not only to psychoanalysis but also to clinical psychiatry, which at least does not publish papers with false postures.

Holzman (1973) wrote that research in psychoanalysis is deficient because of "inadequate clinical training of investigators, poor scientific training in psychoanalytic institutes and a narrow concept of research tasks."

Jurgen Ruesch (1975d) stated: "Improvement of communication is contingent upon recognition that teamwork implements collectively chosen goals, while theorizing and therapeutic skills are learned on an individual basis. Individual attainment of the highest order seems to flourish where professional organization and training stimulate creative activity, minimizing indoctrination of the generation in views and skills which might have outlived their usefulness."

The modern history of psychoanalysis has revealed the enormous shifts in patterns of thinking, moving from an open to a closed system and currently back to an open system. The structural frame of reference and the slow development of adaptational theory has in part been one of the current achievements. We have attempted to move toward a more general biopsychosocial theory, open systems, and transactions involving drives. Yet, there is tremendous resistance to change in theory, thereby blocking the further development of psychoanalysis. In fact, almost all current psychoanalytic issues are not well discussed, but authoritative statements are reiterated as if factual solutions were at hand.

It has been a long time since Freud wrote to Jung: "I am more and more persuaded of the cultural value of psychoanalysis and I could wish for someone bright enough to draw from it the legitimate inferences for philosophy and social life."

We can agree with Frenkel-Brunswick (1952), who states that there are a number of problems that can be solved only by an explicit integration of psychoanalysis with psychology proper and with sociology. The conceptual tools of psychoanalysis are not sufficient to explain fully rational and social behavior.

On the other hand, the biological roots of motivation derived from Freud's early training and incorporated in his "project" have been neglected. Yet, his references to heredity, constitution, and variable strengths of the instincts reveal that Freud maintained the haunting notion that motivation could possibly be derived from biological structure-functions. But these concepts also clearly reveal his adherence to the self-action theory rather than to a continuous interdependence on physiology-in-process, which was no longer significant for psychoanalytic theory, and most persons who attempted to pursue psychophysiological research were considered to be outside the field of psychoanalysis. Any change from the conceptions of psychic energy or cathexis to field concepts, information, or communication theory in another vocabulary was considered as divergence from psychoanalysis.

Despite the germinal influence psychoanalysis has had on psychiatry, psychology, and society and culture, its imperfections have not been corrected nor its truths established by testable hypotheses; changes have been more in the nature of emphasis on its parts by the use of tunnel vision. There has been an irrational resistance to potential and necessary changes in the basic tenets of theory and the standard technics of treatment. Analysts seem to have a narcissistic investment in certainty, as if they fear the loss of their personal organizational integrity. Therefore, basic issues are rarely discussed, and the authoritative elite of the establishment are continuously quoted and reelected to office. Phenomenology is degraded with the implication that clothes (meaning behavior) do not reveal the person.

Wheelis (1956) wrote it well:

> Some analysts who take refuge in dogma become the serious and able defenders of orthodoxy. They are constantly busy maintaining and decorating the house that Freud built, and they openly and honestly oppose anyone bent on remodeling. They may be arch-conservatives, but they have integrity; and what they profess, they believe. Others who make of their science a creed are less successful. They achieve but an uneasy suppression of doubt, and remain divided within. Covertly the doubt spreads. They believe neither in the value of their work nor in the validity of their concepts, but gloss over their disbelief, pretending all is well. Because they do not openly face their misgivings, they suffer an insidious undermining of integrity. They are reactionary in the extreme; yet they defend nothing. They don't study, they don't write, and hence cannot ably support orthodox theory.

Finally, the importance attached to the term *insight,* supposed to differentiate psychoanalysis from other therapies, is not vital because no one can state clearly what it means, how it is acquired, and how long it lasts. Piers (1953) wrote about the lack of human inborn programming so that the child must learn by conditioning to form a superego, by identification to develop an ego-ideal (not imitation), by "insight" to develop the ego.

Psychoanalysis can become a science by using the scientific methods of thinking and operating without sacrificing its conceptual domain or intrinsic methods. There is a great need for it to become an *open system* with freer exchange through its boundaries. Progressive evolution does not occur in isolation, but only through partial separation (specialization) to concentrate the genetic pool (conceptual formation) and by transaction with other groups to add gene symbols (communication) and to test them through natural selection (scientific method). This I hope will be the future course of psychoanalysis.

Roy Schafer (1978) has written a critique of metapsychology, and following Bertalanffy, Ruesch and I have leaned toward general systems theory. Under higher orders of control and regulation, there is partial autonomy, partial subordination, and partial conflict of parts in action. These are functions not reified as exemplified by the phrase "the ego knows" or the "inner surface of the ego." Action occurs by an "I" with an identity, a self, as Martin Buber has stressed. In treatment, the patient becomes conscious of his activity, as against the erroneous view of being passively under control by some inner force.

The *future* is presaged by Robert R. Holt's (Grinker, 1975d) statement: "Much of what Freud had to say is more or less false unless read sympathetically—that is, not with the desire to find him right at all costs but to learn from him."

The future of psychoanalysis, I believe, rests on the abandonment of clichés, fads, and movements; on recognizing the place of psychoanalysis in a general psychiatric system; on observations and descriptions with prediction, reliability, and validation; and follow-up of patients after diagnosis and treatment.

CHAPTER 14

Education

WHATEVER THE FUTURE of our species and our civilization, as responsible psychiatrists we are participants in the process. We should continue to learn, to teach, and to treat patients, families, and groups with the methods that are available to us. In cooperation with our fellow behavioral scientists working in other disciplines, we must participate within the larger scientific community by rendering advice and engaging in social action based on knowledge—we should never be content to promulgate injudicious opinions and absurd generalizations.

Changes in training are not necessarily based on an increase in real knowledge, but rather stem from extensions of responsibility and from the development of new or modified frames of reference and from the experience gained from their practical applications. In large part, graduate education in the clinical training centers attempts to make up what universities and medical schools have neglected or omitted entirely. Such deficits will become even greater and more difficult to offset if the time allotted to education is decreased and the internship is abolished. Instead of the physicians and specialists we need, we will be seeing only immature products of our educational system who are unaware of the meaning of the serious human life problems that they are asked to resolve.

Our dangerous world is changing with an accelerating speed that strains our powers of adaptation. It is hard to know whether the end result will be termed progress by posterity—the validity of such a designation is far from clear. The notion of progress may turn out to be only a coping device that saves us from "giving up" and disintegrating internally. We have been accustomed to viewing man's struggles in this dangerous world—a world in which physical events are less threatening than one's fellow men—from the standpoint of defenses, coping, or adaptation. Goal-seeking behavior is seen as part of the homeostatic mechanism appropriate and economic at a given time, but frequently maintained as neurotic repetition compulsions, despite their success in reducing anxiety. But such a vew of human progress neglects goal-changing behavior as the basis for creativity and change. We are not even sure of the requirements of creativity: Does it need talent, conflict, mastery of crises in the life cycle, or a combination of these factors? Or does it need others that we do not yet understand?

In such a rapidly changing world, it is difficult for those of us who are part of the contemporary social system to predict the character of the psychiatric profession on which future systems of education will be based. Nevertheless, we do know that, because of the sheer numbers of patients we will have to treat and the increasing demands for service, we will have to cooperate and participate in the teaching of psychiatric social workers, clinical psychologists, nurses, and paraprofessionals.

This does not mean that we are sure that what we teach is immutable. What we think we know and teach is for the most part a body of knowledge that only gives us the *illusion* of certainty. We need to create and innovate, to continually check and evaluate. Thus, it is a sad mistake to separate clinical from research programs. Neither can exist alone. We produce psychiatrists and other professionals who are interested in the problems of humans in distress and investigators who know the nature of deviant behavior.

It is also clear that good patient care is not only essential to training but also insures community support. The wide range of therapies that are now in existence must include crisis and brief emergency therapy for members of the community who seek help directly, and they should also serve as a backup for community mental health centers that are concerned with rehabilitation. More emphasis must be placed on limited goals. We must develop a respectable eclectic viewpoint—abandoning nothing, but putting each technique in its proper perspective. Highly articuulated ideologies of specific "schools" should be dismissed—their results have been disappointing. Instead, the focus should be on the "here-and-now" needs of the disturbed or deviant person.

The community psychiatrist, for example, is fulfilling a new role—one requiring an enormous change in perspective for the professional. Gerald Caplan (1961), one of the most influential theorists and educators in this new field, describes the community psychiatrist as different from his traditional colleagues in having to provide services for a large number of people with whom he has had no personal contact, and of whose identity and location he has no initial knowledge. He cannot wait for patients to come to him, because he has equal responsibility for all those who do not come. A significant part of his job consists in finding out who the mentally disordered are and where they are located in his community, and he must deploy his diagnostic and treatment resources in relation to the total group of sufferers, rather than restrict them to the select few who ask or are referred for help.

Additionally, there are federal demands to fulfill. At first, community mental health centers were beneficiaries of a gracious federal largesse, but today their subsidies are being severely threatened. Their programs are involved in serious internal controversy as well. They are criticized for distorting psychiatic training, for embodying the arrogance of social engineering by euphoric experts, for making and breaking extravagant promises to poor and distraught communities, and for serving the political needs of power-seeking federal bureaucrats. To some extent, the program's rise and fall reflects society's suspicion of federal activism in general and the challenges that have risen to many Great Society programs. But just as important, the demise of many such programs throws light on the wavering of the American faith in the power of social environment and in the ability of mental health experts to control and manipulate it.

In delineating the boundaries of modern psychiatry, it is well to remember that the psychiatrist functions solely in the realm of behavioral dysfunction. He is not an expert in dealing with poverty, overpopulation, urban renewal, automation, or war. However, he should be capable of expertly dealing with the behavioral difficulties that *might arise* in people who suffer from deprivation, crowding, slums, unemployment, or massive stress. However tempted he may be to overstep the boundaries of his expertise, the psychiatrist lacks the power to implement social action outside of the mental health field.

In the days when the community mental health clinics were discussed, funded, and put in operation, I spoke out in protest: I knew full well that the boom would eventually be lowered, and less support would be available for the education of mental health professionals. Still, it was no satisfaction to learn of the political turmoil in the communities, of the power struggle initiated by the community members of the committees overseeing the activities of the centers. It was no satisfaction to observe that the centers served as sources of referral to already established institutions in the region. In some places, emergency, crisis, and telephone services were added, but not as effectively as planned. Many psychiatric directors resigned in disappointment, to be replaced by psychologists, social workers, or nurses. Sad to say, the community centers in Chicago only added to the beds of adjacent state hospitals or increased the facilities of favored medical schools. And little more was known about prevention than had been known when the mental hygiene movement first blossomed in the 1920s and failed.

Throughout its long history, as we know, medical education has been directed toward training practitioners to diagnose and treat disease of the body. Students are taught the art of assembling diverse signs and symptoms into meaningful patterns or gestalts, called diseases, for which appropriate statements of course or prognosis can be made and appropriate treatments can be prescribed when known. Interest in causes and prevention has become intensified as natural sequences of events have become recognized. Somehow, medicine became recognized as a scientific view that was facilitated in this country by the Flexner report of 1910.

Dependent on the so-called basic sciences of physiology, biochemistry, pathology, and microbiology, etc., medicine at first was only an applied science, though the direct application of laboratory experimentation to clinical problems could not always be made. Gradually, medicine became the empirical research arm of biological theory.

We are beginning to discover, however, that such a view is only a simplistic notion. The scientific paradigm of holding independent variables steady during experimentation results in the creation of narrow foci, in isolation from other larger systems. Interests became polarized in fundamental elements, reaching down to principles of the physicochemical sciences. Some reductionism squeezes the life of the larger biological organisms. Complex systems falsely come to be seen as linear or single, causal chains of events, and the effects of early and later experiences on the form and function of the organism are neglected. Paradoxically, the trend toward the development of intense interest in psychological and sociological factors that may alter biological functions either temporarily or permanently can also amount to severe distortions in our perception. "Humanism" and "behaviorism" represent a kind of movement toward ideological polarities that is as narrow as reductionist thinking.

It is sobering to realize that we have gained little more knowledge about man in his totality than ancient philosophers such as Aristotle had; only our vocabulary is different. The psychiatrist focuses on human behavior in health and in illness through observations, descriptions, and test challenges for both actions and verbalizations. He realizes that, at a fictitious state of rest or idling, he can observe few significant differences among people sick or well. He also realizes that a sophisticated mode of thinking views behaviors as a conglomerate of allocated functions designated and studied by a number of disciplines. Our goal must be to try to put these all together in a meaningful relationship or organization—to strive toward establishing a unitary theory.

Thomas Mann (1942 to 1949) beautifully articulated this imperative to view man as a whole two decades ago:

> And yet, this is a time and world where it makes almost no difference what we talk about—we always talk about one and the same thing. Categories crumble, the borderlines between the different spheres of human thought become unessential. Everything is connected with everything else—and, in truth, it has always been so: only, we are not conscious of it. Once, it was possible to distinguish between a "purely

> esthetic," "purely philosophic," "purely religious" sphere and the sphere of politics, of human society, of national and international community life and to declare that we are interested in the one but not in the other. This is no longer possible. We are interested in the whole, or we are interested in nothing.

In its trend toward ever finer degrees of specialization, medicine has been especially guilty in viewing the organism in terms of isolated systems, and thus neglecting the human person as a total organization. It is common to blame our "information explosion" as the primary cause of this atomistic focus, but the trend was obvious long ago. We are not only bombarded with more and more information, but an "exchange" has taken place, as past "facts" become untenable and new "facts" are temporarily substituted.

To determine what qualities, skills, and knowledge will equip a psychiatrist to function adequately in a complex and rapidly changing field is no small task. Psychiatrists should have a special appreciation for the negative effects upon a developing mind of a formalized education that sets rigid standards, ideals, and values. In the behavioral sciences, which are so controversial and poorly defined, and where future developments are so hard to predict, such limitations are particularly important to recognize.

It is virtually impossible to agree on the content of a training program, and I am proud to say that our unwillingness at P & PI to formalize or rigidify has been one of the most outstanding achievements of our institute's staff. We have recognized that diverse personalities with different internal psychodynamics, with varying knowledge and experiences, will be the most likely to develop new therapies and original investigations.

We have reached some valuable conclusions, however, through trial and error. First, let me emphasize that a good psychiatrist should also be a good doctor. He must consider the patient's welfare to be primary, and he must vow to do him no harm. He must have a high level of intelligence and an interest in accomplishing beneficial results for others. He must have a sound medical education, and today we can happily rely on most of the American medical schools for this, as well as the general hospitals training our interns. Without the further acquisition of a broad educational background, he cannot be a truly good doctor. He needs to know much about life and living that is not obtainable in a specialized curriculum.

It has been said repeatedly that, in addition to his medical education, the potential psychiatrist should be a warm, sensitive person with an intuitive grasp of hidden feelings and a sincere liking for people. The candidates who seek to be selected for training all tell us that they have these characteristics in correct proportions. To use such characteristics as criteria would be just as bad as to reject candidates on the basis of some nosological diagnostic classification of their particular neuroses. What living being is not to some degree, and sometimes, warm, sensitive, intuitive, and compassionate toward other humans? And, what living person is not to some degree paranoid, phobic, compulsive, homosexual, or depressed? A psychiatrist cannot be defined by his temperature, rate of oxygenation, sensory thresholds, or by his neurosis.

The problem of defining what it is that does make a good psychiatrist is obviously far more complex than that. Let us frame the question in a different way. At what times, in what situations, and to what degree are special forms of communication usable to a person in his attempt to assist another? The selection of potential psychiatrists depends primarily on the recognition of the processes that are necessary for successful functioning in relation to another person. Such processes, we find, are all primarily dependent on various forms of communication. The patient communicates to the psychiatrist; the psychiatrist undergoes a process of internal communication or association and communicates through a feedback mechanism to the patient. Patient and doctor interact in a two-way, circular, *transactional process* within a special environment, each assuming a role pertinent and specific to his position within this process. The result is that the stronger personality, who assumes the role of the physician or the psychiatrist, seeks to have an effect on the sicker personality, who has been assigned by circumstances the role of the weak, dependent, and helpless patient.

To perform the functions assumed in the role of psychiatrist, then, a person must have the capacity to communicate with others. He must know the im- and explicit social roles that his patient enacts and those that are expected of him in transaction with his patient. His skill depends on rapidly shifting the social roles as they are cued by the patient's needs. Equally necessary is the capacity to prevent himself from passively following the cues and commands of the patient; the psychiatrist must thoroughly understand them and must be alert to their internal motivations. Only by remaining distant from overt emotional, relationships with the patient—no matter how tempting—can he press for the patient's understanding of what he is asking for by turning his attention inward.

The second function the potential psychiatrist must perform with endurance communicating successfully with himself. If he has an open system that permits transactions among the various foci within his own personality, he may draw from the codification of his previous experience and feed back to the patient the benefits of a knowledgeable communication that is more than a simple response to a stimulus. This kind of open system or communication with self is often extremely painful. The psychiatrist should be able to recognize many of his own emotions and have the capacity to endure the suffering of feelings such as anxiety, guilt, or depression as they are evoked within him. This ability is particularly hard to evaluate. Health or illness is the end result of a variety of transacting factors, from constitutional structuralization to genetic and current life situations, which may exist in a more or less stabilized state of ease (comfort) or disease (suffering). If health and comfort have been attained at the cost of rigidity or intellectual repression, the flexibility of the psychiatrist is inevitably decreased. If disease or suffering becomes too great, there may be an attendant over- or underevaluation of one's own problems and, therefore, of the patient's suffering.

The third process that seems important to the functioning of a psychiatrist is his integrative capacity—the ability of the intrapsychic transactional systems to maintain themselves as an organization without disintegration under conditions of stress. What external events disturb him, how much he does become disturbed, to what degree or type of equilibrium he returns, and how fast this occurs are parameters of his integrative capacity. These need to be measured not only in terms of the stress the psychiatrist must endure in his own life situations, but also in terms of those stresses patients constantly impose on him. The life of a psychiatrist is especially hard. Though he is constantly bombarded with all sorts of disturbing emotions, he must maintain a stability and equilibrium that are not expected of other professionals—or indeed of other persons.

Finally, the psychiatrist should have a system of personal values derived from the ethnic and cultural influences of his early environment, which is sound and healthy. Such values are expressed in terms of the integrity and incorruptibility of his superego and through the sincere and consistent manner in which he moves toward the realization of his ego ideals. With it all, his values must be flexible enough to adapt to the changing needs and demands of his environment.

There is another aspect to the problem of selection for training of the doctor-psychiatrist that I would like to make clear through an analogy. During World War I, the air force pilots were chosen through no special selection methods. They had no knowledge of scientific aeronautics, but flew by the "seat of their pants." They used their semicircular canals for learning their position in space, their vibratory sense and hearing for knowledge of their machines. Each man developed his own methods and tricks of flying through his own research. The early psychoanalysts also worked by the seat of their pants. They called it intuition, empathy, or "third ear," etc. Each did his own research and published papers concerned with his own tricks and knowledge of certain kinds of dreams and his personally developed techniques.

The first pilots were not as invulnerable as they thought. In fogs, they often flew upside down without knowing it and crashed when visual contact with the land was absent. Analysts, too, were in fogs of the deep unconscious, for they were involved within a single system that constituted an internal function with nothing to "take a fix on." In spite of the resistance of the first pilots, the elements required in flying were finally analyzed and understood, and pilots were subsequently selected with the necessary special aptitudes. Machines were improved to indicate position in time and space, and gauges registered the functioning of the important engines that maintained the ship aloft. Unfortunately, many analysts, like the old pilots, refused to analyze their jobs, to recognize their participant functions and countertransferences, or to use landmarks for time and space.

We have also come to realize that for adequate development of a circular, self-corrective system, the psychiatrist needs to know more than just the psychic system, and the psychoanalyst needs *to understand more than the unconscious.* Both need to know what forces transact with the personality: from the environment on one hand and from the body on the other, for, in varying directions and at various times, both have their impact on the input-output systems of the mental apparatus.

It could be said that psychiatrists and psychoanalysts are practitioners who try to understand the psychosomatic environmental systems as processes in transaction within a particular universe or field. The psychiatrist or analyst is usually interested most intensely in varying levels of the psychic system. The physiologist or physician penetrates into the depths of activities of the somatic system. The sociologist is more concerned with the interaction of individuals as total persons with various social or environmental settings. It has become increasingly clear, as we have suggested, that it is not possible for any person to fully understand a system by working within that system alone. One can learn more about interrelations between somatic and psychic or between psychic and social systems by making observations at the boundaries of their interactions. However, in order to understand more adequately the processes at work in the total psychosomatic-social field, one must understand the processes that occur in transaction among at least three systems from the perspective of one specific field of behavior.

The psychiatrist or psychoanalyst must know the signs of somatic processes effected by the ego as they assume varying social roles in the transactions involving himself and his patient. By doing so, he will not accentuate one aspect of these transactions, nor will he overlook others. He will not be accused of confining his concerns to the lower levels of the unconscious mental processes, nor will he be accused of completely ignoring the effects of reality on the personality or the influences of physical dysfunctions on behavior. Such limited approaches would not require more than the highly specialized knowledge of one discipline. The well-trained psychiatrist needs to know the extent of his own field, the boundaries beyond which he cannot skillfully reach without calling upon professional help from other disciplines.

The transactional principles can only be taught in rudimentary form. The student must learn most of them through his own participation and through his own research. In the selection process, however, we must devise ways of recognizing those who have the potentiality for developing and recognizing transactional communication and weed out those who do not. Those who succeed in meshing these processes with the factual instruction given in any accredited psychiatric training center will find that little that is known about psychiatry or the behavioral sciences will fall into logical and usable operational facets. Practice skills more than knowledge make them competent investigators and masters of a technique that can justifiably be called a science.

Today, there is a growing resistance to psychiatry's penetration into the field of biological, medical, and social sciences. On one hand, there is an extreme attempt to hold back the involvement of psychiatry and psychoanalysis in the study and utilization of somatic processes that have developed in the modern biological sciences. On the other hand, there are indications from within the field as well. Ernest Jones has spoken of the danger of re-reading the findings of psychoanalysis in terms of sociology and has warned of the necessity for unceasing vigilance if such temptations are to be avoided. It is his view that psychoanalysts should observe, study, and try to understand only the inner meaning of surrounding extraordinary events. Such counterreactions to the interest of psychiatry and psychoanalysis in transactional processes (whether they be somatic events or social phenomena) is a gauge of the degree to which *progress is viewed as a threat.*

The point of view I have stressed may be seen more clearly by a formal definition of the psychological system with which psychiatrists and psychoanalysts work in varying depths. The psychological system functions in transaction between the soma, which communicates by means of electrical and chemical signs, and the social and cultural environment, which uses symbolic processes of communication. Through such a process of transaction, the psychological system differentiates, grows, and maintains its functions. Within it, the individual develops varying degrees of awareness or consciousness of the space-time continuum of which he and his species are a part. The psychological system expands in function as a confluence of the projection of all inner and outer surfaces of the organization and its environment.

It is this broad interpretation of psychiatry and this recognition of the necessity of seeing it in its wider social perspective that have guided the process through which we have selected candidates for residencies at P & PI. It was a process that changed and developed through the years, and in all candor I must say that we did not always escape the pitfalls that characterize such enterprises.

Those of us who have the responsibility for selecting candidates for residency in psychiatry continually ask ourselves which applicants should be accepted. After many years of seeing the results of our training programs, we should be better able to judge our criteria, but even now there are too many variables that interfere with making a definitive statement. What are the goals of the training program? What are the goals of the applicant, and how does he or she present himself or herself to each of at least three different interviewers? One research attempt in Chicago to determine the characteristics of the psychiatric residents at all the training centers in a given year failed to discover a consistent pattern.

The applicant always knows what to expect in the interview, because he operates in a fast-moving, national network of communication. Likewise, the interviewers know the standard styles and attitudes of the applicants and judge them somewhat on the places to which they have applied and on the kinds of programs these institutions represent. Little attention is paid to written references or to grades in medical school. The first two years, which largely involve memorizing, are of little relevance to future psychiatrists, and also of little interest, and correspondingly their grades for three years, are apt to be low. Most applicants have little interest in athletics. What is distressing is how little they have read, how little information they have about psychiatry or about the world around them, and how much they lack of intellectual sophistication.

The candidates present themselves as sophisticated people who "like people" and want to "help others." Some are motivated by their own neuroses or by previous illnesses. Many have been influenced by preceptors or by other physicians in the family or within their circle of friends. Many applicants have a missionary spirit, although most of them plan to enter into private practice. Some concede that part-time teaching in a medical school would be acceptable. Only a few are sincerely interested in research and an academic career, and most of those who are, expect to pursue such a course only temporarily. They view psychiatry as a therapeutic field, and have little idea of its past, no feeling for its changing development, and certainly no idea of its extent or of its parts or of their possible future interest in them. In general, their view of psychiatry is no more sophisticated than that of any other member of society.

Although at P & PI we developed a rough rating system, our choices were in effect largely arbitrary. At first we interviewed candidates in groups; later, at the height of the pressure to turn out psychoanalysts, we included the faculty of the analytic institute in the process. Still later we conducted both individual and group interviews, although it was clear that the stress of the group interview situation caused some candidates to break down.

Of course, the real criterion of our success in selection has been the product, and it has varied from year to year. Invariably, we regretted a few of our choices, but more often we were proud of our graduates. In our annual report of 1974 (our twenty-ninth), our institute reported that graduates of our program included nine chairmen of departments, ten professors, twenty associate professors, thirty-one assistant professors, and seven instructors. Many others were engaged in successful private practices with part-time teaching affiliations.

Franz Alexander's academic ambitions had led him to pursue closer ties between the analytic institute and the psychiatric training centers. He envisaged analysis as the focal point for all training. But Henry Brosin, then of the University of Chicago, and I saw otherwise, and, in an effort to engage the training resources in the city in a meaningful collaboration, we finally set up the Associated Psychiatric Facilities. Selection of residents and analytic candidates was carried out through group interviews that included representatives of all the training institutions. Acceptance meant matriculation in analysis, as well as a psychiatric residency. A few "strong" candidates were given rotating residencies at the University of Chicago, the University of Illinois, and Michael Reese Hospital. After a few years, however, this system collapsed because of the difficulties involved in carrying out such a complex arrangement.

A later proposal by the analytic institute to furnish teachers to the residency programs (a means of increasing their own enrollment) was rejected out of hand because most of the residents preferred to learn the principles of psychodynamics from their own teachers (mostly analysts) rather than to enroll in the first-year courses at the institute.

Our educational program at P & PI has been detailed in Chapter 4. Along with our successes, we made some major mistakes in our planning, and it has regrettably taken at least a decade of struggle to undo them. I refer particularly to our struggle for eclecticism, which was the result of an effort to compensate for our error in overemphasizing the principles and methods of psychoanalytic psychiatry. As a kind of counterpoint to the trend toward greater consideration of biological and pharmacological advances, we have moved from clinical studies of the patient-therapist dyad to the larger units (family, group, social, and cultural, etc.).

One of the greatest difficulties in broadening the psychiatric vistas of each individual resident is the highly indigenous language surrounding specific theories. Language, it must be remembered, is not an artificially learned instrument, but represents modes of thinking and conceptual formulations. If one can induce the resident to learn the meaning of the transactional, the sociological, the communicational, and the informational processes both conceptually and operationally, he will be able to use the appropriate language for each aspect of modern psychiatry. Since at the present time we have few transformational hypotheses and must view each conceptual system independently or translate one into another by substituting words, it is difficult to achieve a thorough understanding of theoretical differences.

Another critical problem is the need of the student for security and certainty and the wish to participate in a field where statements can be made with some assurance regarding what is known and what should be done. Such a need can be met in the field of psychiatry only through the rigid formulations and stereotypes commonly promulgated by the unscientific followers of Freud, who assert that they are following "our science." Such a statement is, of course, a paradox in itself, because a science can belong to no one. Such possessiveness only indicates an attitude of rigidity and complacency and can only be injurious to the developing psychiatrist. We must continually challenge, test, and indicate alternative hypotheses, to make the student aware that there are aspects of psychiatry other than the psychodynamics and frames of reference other than the psychoanalytic.

I believe this points to a new direction for a curriculum of education that, as can be seen from this outline, is multidisciplinary and not entirely medical. Some of it should be incorporated in the university, some in the premedical years, but much of it, however, is medical; at least, it is a continuous process. The real purposes are to give to the student a concept of the totality of the life cycle, the transactional relationship among its parts, the components of the parts, and to avoid reductionism on the one hand and "existentionism" on the other. If we could give this full picture and then fill in the details, not only with contributions from scientific disciplines but also by the specialties of the applied medical sciences, then, even though there are a variety of approaches and differences of methods, the total picture could give meaning to a concept of all of life, containing so-called healthy and sick components. This is an example of unitary thinking.

Within the medical specialties compartmentalized in named departments, there are "core areas" that need to be taught and within which experience by practice is necessary for adequate mastery, no matter whether the product mounts the academic ladder or contentedly exists as a dispenser of services in city or county, singly or in groups. There is, however, another core area basic to the education of all graduate students, no matter what the specialty or what apparent career goals may be favored at the moment. This is a knowledge of the health-illness system, which cannot be fractured, since it denotes a process in continuity over time, i.e. life.

CHAPTER 15

Research

A REMARK by a child psychiatrist whom I was once interviewing on tape epitomized the inability of some professionals to recognize the continuing need for research: "We know everything we need to know about children," he said. "The only problem is how to implement our knowledge." This remark revealed a serious misunderstanding of the nature and the challenges of the psychiatric enterprise. Only by constant testing, evaluation, and study—and only by the continuous sharing of our results—can we sustain our work effectively and move it forward.

It is not easy, however, to select and train an investigator with a critical curiosity directed to humans in distress and the ability to abstract from observed empirical phenomena and creatively seek out problems and persevere in the attempts to solve them.

Even with the appropriate skills and personal qualities, the aspirant for a career in psychiatric research needs nurturing by competent teachers—research models who encourage, advise, and facilitate early experiences and publications. The future psychiatric researcher needs clinical training and experiences and an opportunity to study relevant clinical problems, especially in a multidisciplinary group. At least, the future researcher needs to understand current advances in diagnosis and classification and the importance of framing the right questions.

The techniques of clinical research in psychiatry include observations of behavior, interviews, tests, questionnaires, and follow-up procedures. Even the most competent psychoanalyst must make inferences from the observation of behavior. Any research program must include planning, pilot studies, and eventually a recorder and a statistical analyst. Nevertheless, the best research must not include too much at one time: It should use only a fragment of the general systems theory of a larger program if it is to be a single, well-focused project. In the book *Psychiatry in Broad Perspective* (1975, pp. 97-99), I have quoted a checklist of questions for research programs R.R. Holt, originally published in *Experimental Methods in Clinical Psychology*. Conversely, the current approach, employed in *The Borderline Syndrome* (Grinker, Werble, and Drye, 1968b), translates ego-functions into observable behaviors.

During the planning and pilot stages of a research project, there is always excitement, but since modern clinical research is lengthy and arduous—six months to several years—boredom inevitably ensues until the period of data analysis brings renewed enthusiasm. The researcher often encounters (and must struggle with) clinicians hostile to the use of their clinical material for research.

Long experience in clinical and multidisciplinary research has taught me how poor initial planning can sabotage a research program. The multiple disciplines composing psychiatric science make problems of integration difficult. The postwar psychodynamic model has been seriously confronted by the biological model on the one hand and by sociology, medical economics, politics, and community psychiatry (with its increasing consumerism) on the other. There is just too much for the scientific psychiatrist to know well—it is no wonder that the spirit of inquiry and the skepticism about so many parts of the field have become strained. Few research psychiatrists are being trained to learn both the "hard" neurological and the "soft" sociobehavioral sciences. Three areas of psychiatric training and research are especially weak: evaluation research, research in child psychiatry, and research on the etiology of nonpsychotic disorders, e.g. neuroses and character disorders, etc.

There are indications that the most able students who are grounded in the sciences are not going into the study of medicine and that few of the most competent young physicians are choosing psychiatry as a specialty. Our formal and informal efforts to recruit researchers from the existing pool of young psychiatrists should be intensified. There is a need for the academic professor of psychology and the teacher of psychiatry to set before his students in the first two years of medicine the possibilities and the rewards of a satisfactory research career in the mental health field. It is by increasing the intellectual level of aspiring doctors that we may hope to develop productive investigators.

Zubin (1952, 1972) points out that a suitable research model would be a reconstruction of nature to use in studying a given phenomenon. The model simplifies nature in order to facilitate research. A current example is a computer that analogizes systems of communication disturbances with psychopathology. Zubin states that there are six models in psychiatry: ecological, developmental, learning, hereditary, internal environment, and neurophysiologic. Not only these models but the interaction among them must be studied.

How does a private hospital develop a research program? Without funds from a parent university or a substantial endowment, the private hospital must either rely on its own meager income or turn to granting agencies or local philanthropists. Though it is often said that research grants are given only to hospitals with academic affiliations, this is not the case (Oken et al. 1962).

The specific problems that a hospital chooses to study grow naturally out of the *clinical questions* it faces. There is no dearth of these. The investigator begins by formulating hypotheses and then tries to narrow them down through observation. He develops and tries out techniques appropriate to the detailed measurement and observation of the phenomena. Next, he outlines an appropriate research design for a formal investigation. Informal observations thus grow first into pilot studies and then into more controlled, specific research projects. Eventually, a broad program of interrelated studies may evolve.

Uncomplicated short-term projects that can be approached directly with the natural tools of clinical observation represent a logical first step in developing a research program. Extensive global investigations that might never get finished should be avoided. The resources, limitations, and special features of the institution, including personnel, physical plant, patient population, and available staff time, must all be taken into account.

Factors that may initially appear to be obstacles to private-hospital research may in fact be assets. The private hospital's lack of administrative superstructure may actually enhance its flexibility. There is no dean or legislative committee to "suggest" or approve projects. The primary responsibility of the hospital is to treat a relatively small number of patients—a role that makes possible painstaking, intensive clinical observations. Individualized treatment permits comparisons of various approaches. The higher socioeconomic level of the patients reflects, to some extent, their previous success in adapting and, therefore, their personality strengths, affording a closer view of the positive integrative forces of personality organization. Certain diagnostic entities, for example, depressions and character disorders, are more common and thus more accessible to study. Because most private hospitals have many close ties with the patient's home, illness and treatment can be studied on a continuing basis within the patient's natural family and social setting.

These considerations clearly point to the fact that clinical research is the forte of the private psychiatric hospital. Though complex laboratory experiments may fascinate the neophyte in these days of scientific breakthroughs, basic research should be initiated only after the private hospital has achieved some success in clinical studies. Ideally, laboratory investigations focus on questions growing out of clinical studies. But it may be years before a private hospital is ready to undertake laboratory research, if, indeed, ever.

Other institutions, particularly universities, have excellent laboratories for basic research, but good clinical research remains at a premium. Moreover, clinical research costs much less than basic research, because it does not require expensive, quickly obsolescent equipment.

Almost every private psychiatric hospital can contribute valuable knowledge if it focuses on problems commensurate with its resources and clinical problems (Oken et al., 1962). Neither a huge budget nor superscientific gadgets are needed. The main essentials are curiosity, motivation, and open communications between patient-subjects and physician-observers. In addition, it is necessary to plan carefully and to work slowly through each necessary stage, using sound scientific principles, without permaturely rushing into global programs. The greatest dangers lie in trying to solve complex problems through elaborate research without first dealing with more basic issues and in overemphasizing the role of the laboratory.

In P & PI's hospital-institute, we have carried out a number of research projects. The development of each illustrates the value of starting out simply, then proceeding to more complex studies. The scope of the studies illustrates the wide range of projects a privately supported center can undertake. These resulted in many papers on stress, anxiety, and psychophysiological responses (Grinker et al., 1950-1957) .

One research project involved a social science research group comprising three sociologists, a social psychologist, and a member of the full-time psychiatric staff. This group was able to delineate a much more explicit picture of different psychiatric attitudes or "ideologies" and develop quantitative scales to assess these philosophies. It then explored, by direct observation, the effects of the different ideologies upon diagnoses and treatments (Strauss et al., 1964) .

Other basic studies included neuroendocrine relationships, the neurophysiology and neuropsychology of specific brain areas, especially the limbic system, and biochemical processes in the brain. Ideas or suggestions arising from this work are explored in the stress laboratory or on the wards, to clarify their relevance to human function. Thus, clinical and basic studies cross-fertilize each other. But the keystone of our work is clinical research.

It is clear that, without a profound understanding of human psychopathology, all other disciplines involved in psychiatry, such as genetics, biochemistry, and sociology, dangle free without the support of stable referrents.

On the other hand, psychiatrists are notoriously *poor observers of behavior.* Their training has usually emphasized the importance of listening to verbal statements in order to understand covert meaning. Clinical psychologists, on the other hand, observe well, and when reporting shifts in unstructured tests, describe in great detail the behaviors of their subjects.

It may seem that the tools of clinical research are possessed by anyone with eyes, ears, and a capacity for abstraction, but this is far from true.

Conducting *interviews* requires both the patience to listen to unstructured communications and the ability to develop subsequent structured interrogations that reflect a knowledge of sequences of thinking and feeling appropriate for the goal of the specific research. Interviewing is a delicate tool that needs complete familiarity with the goal of the study, continuity in its use to acquire a body of experience, and sensitivity to the patient's feelings and defensive maneuvers. This skill is not easily perfected and, like any instrument, it needs constant calibration.

Questionnaires are not simple instruments that can be put together quickly. They need considerable thought to be sure that their items are directly pertinent to the information sought. Furthermore, each word needs to be carefully studied to be sure that it has a universally and well-understood single meaning. For example, in one investigation, a question asked college students was worded: "Was your mother concerned about ____?" The word "concern" was interpreted by some as *worried* and by others as benign *interest*. To avoid such indefinite questions, the questionnaire should be pretested widely.

Questionnaires must be constructed to fit the goals of each research project and cannot be borrowed. For example, in studying the predisposition to the development of operational fatigue (war neuroses) by flying personnel (Harrower and Grinker, 1946), we devised a "stress tolerance test"—a new projective technique, utilizing both meaningful and meaningless stimuli, which furnished an objective measure of the degree of the subject's improvement. Another special technique was devised to produce anxiety by perceptual distortion in order to determine its threshold (Basowitz et al., 1955).

Although clinical research is primarily carried on by psychiatrists and clinical psychologists, other investigators in the mental health field, such as social workers, anthropologists, and sociologists, often participate as well.

Only recently has the psychologist become an equal and integral part of the research team. Although psychiatrists were accustomed to ordering psychologists to perform psychological tests as if they were laboratory technicians, gradually the clinical psychologist has insisted on being a consultant to the psychiatrist before and after his psychometric activities were carried on. Both groups have recognized that psychological tests must be specially adapted to the goals and parameters of each research program and must be continually reevaluated and redesigned.

Both the psychologist and the psychiatrist have learned from each other; the clinical psychologist has become less interested in specific tests for psychopathology and has relied more on the interview, and the psychiatrist too has learned greater skills in engaging in an interview and in interpreting it. The psychoanalytic intrusion of the last several decades has had an impact on both professions, and the strong biological emphasis has become somewhat mitigated.

Psychologists have unquestionably made a significant contribution to research, though psychology is not the basic science of psychiatry in the way that physiology is basic to medicine. Psychologists have an interest, of course, in the drive theories from which psychopathology is presumed to develop. Thus, for example, increased stimulus input, acting on a heightened drive arousal, would be accompanied by a low threshold for disorganization and stimulus generalization. An inadequately modulated system, therefore, requires narrowed attention as a protective device if input is to be reduced and excessive excitation is to be avoided.

Constructs such as Rimoldi's innate logical structures, Piaget's ontogeny of thought, Vogotsky's development of inner speech as a problem of social psychology, and Whorf's studies on language, thought, and reality have made a significant contribution to psychiatric research.

About the value of hypnosis as a tool with which to probe into the depths of personality, there is considerable uncertainty. The adequacy of evidence from various experiments that have been carried on is in doubt, and the concepts of hypnosis are still not clearly defined.

A psychiatric institute such as P & PI contains other kinds of research laboratories as well: laboratories of neurophysiology, neuropsychology, and biochemistry. All contribute to a better understanding of the totality of the processes of health and illness in man. Embedded within a psychiatric institute, experimental scientists contribute to and receive from the clinicians more than they could in isolation, because each group is constantly in contact with others and thus learns the problem questions, the methodological limitations, and the tests for appropriateness.

In general, such research activities are directed toward the understanding of the neurophysiological and neuroendocrinological mechanisms underlying behavior and experience. Since mental illnesses revolve around disturbances of affect, learning, memory, and perception, these are the psychological categories on which attention must be focused.

The P & PI laboratories are equipped to study the behavior of a variety of species, including rats, cats, monkeys (including the recently discovered docile stump-tailed monkey), and man. Neuropsychological methods include ablation, electrical stimulation, and the recording of bioelectrical potentials of the brain (Giannitrapani, 1974). Behavior is manipulated by imposing conditions of deprivation of enrichment on the organism. Various tests are applied to study discrimination, sensory capacities, memory, and emotion.

The involvement of our psychophysiological theory in human research is exemplified by the use of the Necker cube, a reversible image, to study human perception and to observe processes of satiation from which laws of neurophysiological processes are being derived. A new instrument, the adjustable body-distorting mirror, has been invented to measure objectively the human's self-body image and its distortions. Since *psychiatric and neurological disorders* are often accompanied by distortions in body image, there is reason to hypothesize that they may be primary to the development of ego distortions. These are significant indicators, causes, or results of the most malignant psychiatric disturbances, such as schizophrenia.

There have also been extensive studies of *the anatomical substrate* of psychological functions in the brain. Using such methods as selective stimulation and destruction of discrete anatomical regions of the brain, some success has been achieved in this effort. This has encouraged us to ask whether a similar relationship exists between drug localization and action. Although pharmacological action may involve more than drug localization in a specific area, it is pertinent to know the pattern of entry, the mechanism of penetration through the blood-brain barrier, the distribution, and localization of drugs in the various parts of brain, as well as their disposition. Only when such information is available for a large number of centrally acting drugs are we in a position to evaluate the relationship between regional localization and drug action and to develop a true psychopharmacology (Nair, 1964).

Other biological studies have been published from time to time by other institutes, but are rarely verified. Williams (1956) relates constitution to specific personalities. His formula is: Genes give rise to enzymes that create various nutritional needs, such as alcoholism. Sheldon (1973) correlated body build, derived from an intricate series of measurements, with personality and temperament, etc. Brain-damaged persons, with their catastrophic reactions, anxiety, and concrete thinking, have been compared with similar findings in schizophrenics.

Activities of the nervous system have been dichotomized into reflex and learned behaviors, not inborn and not specified by the gene pattern. To understand learned behavior, ethologists have studied early imprinting on experimental animals. The field is highly controversial, and its application to man has not yet been verified.

I have indicated some aspects of psychiatric research in general, but there are many more, since in the field there are many subdisciplines and many methods, all or any of which may contribute to our future understanding of mental illness. However, as Vale

(1973) states: "The major question is how does the genotype or the resulting biochemical processes combine with the environment to produce the behavioral process?"

As a young child, my grandson had an insatiable curiosity about the fascinating world of which he is a part and an intense drive to master its complexities. But he has always had a practical mind as well, for he continually asks when he confronts a new thing, "What do we do with it?" How can I say to him that the true scientist is supposed to be curious without reference to purpose or utility? I would lose his trust, and he would likely reject the career of fourth-generation Grinker psychiatrist!

Native intelligence has transcended the scientific taboo against "teleological causation" when my grandson asks the commonsense questions "what for" or "why." He is supported by C.J. Herrick (1956), who states, "In natural processes there is no dissociation of things and their properties, matter and energy, mechanisms and what they do, organs and their functions, human bodies and human experience, or mind and the setup of objective conditions upon which it is contingent."

"What do we do with it?" is a difficult question, harder to answer than in our presophisticated days of direct clinical impressions. The finest statistical analyses of dozens of traits deal with subtleties that seem to have no clinical reference; those that include only a few cruder measurements tell the clinician little that he does not know already. What seems to be lacking are proper questions derived from empirical experience with human behavior.

Few would object to the laboratory scientist investigating his time and energy in what pleases him or satisfies his desire for play. Who can tell what he will discover or of what use it will be? Yet, there is growing doubt among money-giving agencies of the meaning of research that is related only to personal values. It seems clear, however, that we should insist that clinical research be specifically related to human problems of adaptation in health or illness—to the adjustment, as Herrick (1956) puts it, of the organism to existing conditions. "It is a time-linked process with a past reference and a future reference." Active search should be made "for the mechanisms of this forward reference of adaptive behavior and human purposive behavior." Then only will our experimental technology and our statistical sophistication be applied to significant problems.

For a long time, the nature-nurture dichotomy separated the biological and the psychological disciplines, and to some extent it still does, especially since many American psychoanalysts focus exclusively on psychogenesis. We should remember what Freud wrote about the neuroses: "They are severe, constitutionally fixed illnesses, which rarely restrict themselves to only a few attacks, but persist as a rule over long periods or throughout life." He further stated that we have neglected the constitutional factor in our therapeutic practices. Perhaps we can do nothing about it, but in theory we ought to bear it in mind.

There are indications, however, that biological factors are increasingly being considered in the formulations of etiology of mental disturbances and that concern is growing about the way in which genetics and environmentally induced experiences are interlocked. Rainer (1973) states, "More than a static combination of two factors added together, the interaction is a continuous process with mutual feedback, and spiral development through a series of critical stages."

The extensive investigations on correlations between somatic processes and mental phenomena that have been conducted for over several decades have not, in fact, advanced our thinking much more than those ascribed to Aristotle. The highly acclaimed "breakthrough" originated by Alexander in Chicago into the understanding of the causes of a variety of degenerative diseases by ascribing a specific emotional etiology to each, has been disappointing. As a result, psychosomatic research focusing on specific syndromes has been superseded by renewed psychophysiological investigations, enhanced by modern instrumentation, into the phenomena of relationships between mind and body. These are concentrating mainly on emotions and on autonomic and endocrine functions.

Unfortunately, these relationships cannot be reduced to the desired simplicity by considering somatic processes to be in the service of internal regulation and maintenance within homeostatic boundaries and by considering the mental to be concerned with the outer adaptation of total behavior to events, things, and other living objects. There are several reasons for this major difficulty: The inner-outer dichotomy breaks down operationally; the temporal characteristics of and within each system are widely different; and the mental is not examinable as a form of energy. The following points make this explicit:

1. Inner regulation consists not only of reactions to outer stimuli, but also of responses to inner pressures and motivations leading to *goal-seeking behavior.* In addition, tension states are restlessly *sought* and facilitate *goal-changing behavior* as the basis of change, creativity, and human evolution. These, in turn, require shifts in internal regulation. "In" and "out" are as inseparable as man and his environment.

2. The temporal characteristics of mental operations are as rapid as neural conduction, whereas other somatic processes, such hormonal processes.

Correspondingly, some of these processes occur later than those on which their sequence depends. Obviously, many somatic events become evident long after the psychological stimuli have apparently been dissipated, making correlations difficult if not impossible.

There is no question, as Hamburg has pointed out, that psychiatry is one of the behavioral sciences and that it is concerned with acts of living organisms under specified conditions. All acts have meanings, and all actors respond to both ex– and internal stimuli. Whether the focus of observation is on a single organism or on groups of varying sizes, all have a past that, to some degree, determines their present. No matter how far antecedent or "basic" that past may be, the maturation of any genotype is influenced by environmental conditions.

In the processes of development, action appears first and undergoes successive phases of change. Systems of action at first are global self-actions arising from within. They later become interactional in that one behavior influences another in a linear chain. Finally, action becomes transactional in the sense that reverberatory feedback mechanisms institute control. At the same time, global or undifferentiated behavior becomes more discrete and differentiated. With the ontogeny of complex acts, there is a broadening of the scope of sensory and perceptive systems facilitating even more control. The mediating mechanisms reside in the differentiating functions of the central nervous system.

The various sciences significantly involved in understanding behavior constitute a vast array of disciplines that today cannot be mastered by one person or any reasonably sized group, but all of them should be recognized as extremely important for some aspect of behavior.

The scientific disciplines involved in the total field at times seem to represent irreconcilable viewpoints. This conglomeration, embracing practically the entire field of human transactions, is spoken of as *psychiatry* only for lack of an adequate term to express it. Indeed, each of the behavioral sciences represents an organized pattern of viewing man, using special concepts, methods, and evaluations. Each views behaviors in a special context from a specific frame of reference. Such differences should not be minimized, because each system under study possesses processes regulated by somewhat different invariants.

The above brief statements seem to indicate profound divergencies in theory and method, but they need not be so interpreted. Measurements of behavior in natural or under experimental conditions, *as well as* self-reports, which we have found in the emotional field to be highly reliable, are each appropriate methods for studying various problems, providing the setting and the frame of view of the observer are clearly stated as part of the data requiring analysis. Instincts or drives, emotions and defenses, partial and total behavior, and verbalizations are data suitable for analysis if they are obtained by open and replicable methods and are used to interact with explicitly stated theory. There is no objection to the use of hypothetical constructs or intervening variables, as long as operations are linked to defined referrents and validity is tested by other kinds of operations.

Perhaps merely the recognition that there can be no psycho–, socio–, or somatogenesis *alone* constitutes progress. First, by virtue of their past, all systems—genic or genetic—are prepared for variable responses, both patterned or structuralized, as well as novel and adaptive, to new situations. Second concepts of crude linearity have to be abandoned, since in nature most transactions are curvilinear. Third, causality as an explanation is superseded by concepts of threshold and by the temporal and quantitative properties of a wide range of responses in which the end point may vary with changing conditions and may be the result of a variety of intermediate processes (equifinality). The common final pathway may be reached through a number of diverse processes.

Depending on the drives and needs of the organism and the changing environment, stimuli constantly entering the central nervous system, derived from meaningful environmental cues, set off psychosomatic responses in appropriately sensitive individuals. Depending upon the somatic and psychological sensitivity of the individual, the nature and intensity of the stimulus, the quality of the protective devices, and the psychological defenses available, greater quantities of disturbance lasting for long periods of time (sometimes shorter, as in bereavement) may end in so-called psychosomatic diseases. The ultimate application of this research is to determine the pathways to this end point of illness.

The crucial focus for a consideration of the preparation for health or illness is in the early period of transition in infancy from global, relatively undifferentiated behavior to discrete, differentiated, functional parts of the total system. The impact of the environment, mostly maternal, influences the patterned processes of both soma and psyche.

Some research may be conducted in naturalistic settings in which subjects may carry on their usual behavior, as in anthropological and sociological investigations or in psychiatry on anxiety and stress. Other human investigations employ the experimental method: Stress may be applied in an interview, or motion pictures may be viewed with concomitant or subsequent biochemical, physiological, or psychological tests. Nevertheless, many experimental designs, such as the two mentioned above, are not now feasible because of new requirements for "informed consent."

Another decision that has to be made concerns the use of cross-sectional versus longitudinal approaches, though in certain cases both may be employed. Both approaches have been used in a study of normal adolescents and are being used in our schizophrenic programs. Each approach—cross-sectional and longitudinal—has its place in psychiatric research, but continued follow-up studies are necessary to control in spontaneous or life-experienced changes in the syndrome and shifts in symptoms, as for example in the change from acute to chronic and chronic to terminal schizophrenia.

Follow-up studies in longitudinal research are necessary not only because of changes occurring in different phases of ontogenetic development, but because of the shifting motivation of the subjects and alterations in their patterns of defense and coping, with changing life stresses. In some conditions, outcome depends on the kind and quantity of external social support: for example, for single schizophrenics without a family network as contrasted with those fully accepted and helped by concerned relatives and communities. The follow-up studies may be conducted by interviews, questionnaires, tests, or by a combination of methods. Since the attrition or dropout rate of subjects is often great, and beginning number of subjects should be at least double those expected to cooperate to completion, and the follow-up tactics need to be aggressively pursued.

What kind of *controls* are necessary? First, the same procedures on subjects suffering from conditions different from those under investigation are used. Secondly it is necessary to study so-called normals or healthy persons. These are both difficult to define and difficult to find. In fact, paid volunteers are often psychopathic. In my own work I was successful in studying a group of 134 young adult college males who were psychologically healthy. When I questioned them fourteen years later I found them to be in even better condition than at the time of the first study. Material on these subjects is available for use by any interested investigator (Grinker, 1962, 1963b).

In clinical research, as in any other scientific endeavor, tests for reliability and validity insure the legitimacy of the results, but these can only be expressed in probabilistic terms. The conclusions of the research may be expressed in the hard, firm language of the data obtained, but they may also include new hypotheses and speculations as to their meaning, providing each is clearly defined.

In the study of a human being, unlike research on laboratory animals, there are many uncontrollable factors that, at least, should be recognized. We know that the setting of the research is limited by time and that many extraneous experiences cannot be controlled, even with patients in a hospital ward. What life crises are outside our knowledge? What spontaneous shifts in the disturbance occur? In the here-and-now interview or test procedure, a sample of cognitive, affective, and behavioral structures is obtained, but past histories indicating prior ego strength or predisposing factors are hard to elicit truthfully from the subject or his family.

When dealing with large samples of subjects, in order to wipe out individual differences, a *statistician* should be included in the research team during the planning stages. Sophisticated clinical research today demands more than simple correlational analyses. Instead, cluster, principle component, and/or factor analyses should be employed. All these demand mathematical and statistical expertise that clinicians do not usually possess.

It is crucial, however, that statistical results be matched closely with clinical experience. As clinicians, we have the responsibility of choosing which statistical groupings are logically compatible with clinical experience and that have the optimum degree of discrimination for clinical practice. Frequently a fit that would not have been possible by clinical scanning or statistical analysis alone is achieved.

Using the family as a focus for research, instead of the individual, through observations, interviews, tests, and group tasks may clarify the systems of communications and the power of hierarchy that is crippling at least one of its members.

Aside from the traditional theories developed by psychiatrists and psychologists, a number of mystical concepts that do not offer tools for research are being witnessed. They are phenomenological, dealing only with consciousness and a subjective frame of reference that cannot be altered by commands. Some of these involve the existentialist, who deals with "becoming," the personal construct theory of anticipation of events, the positive self-regard concepts, the "third force" of growth *as* safety, and the search for security. These may be humanitarian in outlook, but they reject objectivity, reality, and research.

A neglected area of research in psychiatry is concerned with development within and among the phases of the life cycle. Certainly there is a patchwork quilt of theories of child development expressed in behavioral terms. Schemas of intelligence as action patterns leading to accommodation to the environment and internalized assimilation have been widely acclaimed. Various serious nutritional, metabolic, infectious, and environmental factors influence future development. Early upsets at environmental changes in infancy may be predictive of later trouble, but the crying need in this field is for longitudinal studies. Studies of the teenager may be systematic and methodologically sound, as contrasted with anecdotal reports of experiences of children.

There seem to be no limits to the extent of biological investigations or how far they may become significant for psychiatry. Restrictions on support for such investigations should not be based on the need for so-called relevance to the human condition: Even *futurologists* constituting a new "science" cannot predict what laboratory, test, or field observations may hold the key to unlock the mysteries of human psychoses. Their usual generalization is, in essence, "More of the same and better than." Irrelevance is a contemporary judgment that may be correct or incorrect, stimulating or depressing future activities.

CHAPTER 16

Current Issues in Psychiatry*

SINCE MY resignation in 1976 as chairman of the Department of Psychiatry and director of the Institute for Psychosomatic and Psychiatric Research and Training, which I opened in 1951 at Michael Reese Hospital and Medical Center, I have been asked to predict the future of psychiatry, to which I have only alluded in the preceding chapters of this book. It is easy enough to make predictions dependent on available money, space, and personnel, ignoring the need for fresh ideas and strategies. I think I have indicated clearly the negative attitudes now existing in the public and nonpsychiatric professional environments. How, then, can one predict the future of a beleaguered field, except to outline hopes for the future?

The *future* of psychiatry obviously depends on the development of research in the field, which sadly needs intensive investigation. Increased knowledge in the field of psychiatry, however, can only be achieved through increased sophistication in research designs and in theoretical concepts. There is no longer room for superficial correlations, which have satisfied us heretofore. Indeed, the complications are so great that young persons interested in investigative careers often turn aside when they contemplate the intracacies of working in a field concerned with human mentation and behavior. The complications of human personalities, their high degree of variability, and the tremendous difficulties in holding parameters constant indeed produces considerable frustration.

---

*This chapter contains a partially abbreviated and modified verson of a paper presented at the two-hundredth anniversary of the Williamsburg State Psychiatric Hospital in West Virginia, October 10, 1973 Courtesy of Dr. George Kriegman.

If we now look again, at the vast area psychiatry now covers, without even being able to guess how much further it will extend, since psychiatry seems to be as broad as life itself, we find divisions based on a number of points of view or orientations. We can recognize easily (1) the orientation of age, which divides psychiatry into the seasons of humans: children, adolescents, adults, and the aging. Some frames of reference (2) are problem-oriented, such as disease classifications, behavioral manifestations, and dynamic or psychoanalytic concepts. These are three approaches that deal with specific problems from separate frames of reference. There is then (3) the action-oriented psychiatry, which is concerned with the study of epidemiology and social engineering. Its prime purpose is that of changing a society, so that its people will not suffer from frustrations and conflicts that end in sickness. Finally, there is (4) an approach-oriented division, which can be divided into the biological, psychological, and the social. Sometimes these are linked together in one biopsychosocial approach.

The variety of these dimensions often has expressed itself in a conflict of either-or. Sometimes this is resolved by the adoption of a reductionistic frame of reference and sometimes by a humanistic frame of reference, indicating that such polarities are often considered quite separate. On the other hand, some attempt to resolve conflict of this nature by the development of general or unified theories, of which general systems theory is one and transactionalism either a part of it or another. These global theories, however, are not operational and often serve as escape hatches. The umbrella of a general theory only encompasses other less global and smaller theories, each of which may contribute to hypotheses requiring well-designed operational research.

In my opinion, we have to recognize restrictions in what we are capable of doing with our limited space and funds and with those investigators whom we can attract. It may be that some of these overlap within our departments. If they are duplications, then they should be allocated to one place or another. If they do not replicate, but show some indication of variance in approach, I see no reason why they cannot be independently prosecuted. I think that special functions in the vast field of psychiatry cannot be allocated a priori, nor can final decisions be made as to where what is done.

Earlier, in Chapter 4, I briefly discussed the issues in the field of psychiatry that obstructed or, at least, were not helpful in developing a scientific psychiatry and interfered with its progress. This became clear even before our new institute at Michael Reese Hospital was built. Not only did I have to struggle for its building and development, but I had to fight to keep it open. I had already been sensitized to such a conflict at the University of Chicago, where I lost the battle, as did the medical school (for three decades). But commitment and hard work gave me freedom, staff excellence, and loyalty, as well as funds for our development at Reese. Thus, as I write about current problems and issues that became too much for me after twenty-five years of service, it is without complaint; I only worry how the present administration will fare.

In this closing golden era of financial support from federal and state governments, new issues seem to arise continually. These absorb the energies of leaders in the field, as service, teaching, and research are affected adversely. The issues are too numerous to receive more than mention.

The medical schools' internships have become poorer; the chronic mental patient has been exiled to psychiatric ghettos; intergenerational conflicts have increased; subclassifications of schizophrenias, psychopathies, and depressions have been neglected; evaluation of the courses of illnesses have spanned too short a time; and evaluations of various forms of treatment are primitive.

I have previously mentioned some of the issues confronting the advance of psychiatry briefly: competing encounter groups giving use to morbidity; psychologists' demands for medical equality; malpractice suits and high insurance premiums; unorganized community psychiatry; splintering of the entire field into small segments; confidentiality; lack of evaluation of all forms of treatment; false notions of prevention; social science blundering into psychiatry; lack of funds; poor quality of psychiatric research and controls; and direction and interference by central regulatory bodies, creating time-consuming wasteful paperwork. Some of these are mentioned in greater detail, as they have grown out of all proportion.

I shall summarize some of the issues—as well as our successes and failures—thus pointing the way, it is hoped, to further advancement in the cause of mental health. Although the psychiatrists are concerned with human beings on an intimate personal level and to a large extent have resisted work in the public health bureaucracy as physicians and social engineers, we must always be mindful of our wider social responsibilities. It is psychiatrists who must know and understand what political and social conditions are conducive to sound mental health or to illness, even though as a profession there is little we can do to create favorable social conditions.

I first became acquainted with the word *psychopolitics* (a term described by James Cavenaugh, Jr., in a recent paper (1978)) during my second term as president of the Illinois Psychiatric Society. The paperwork was so horrendous that there was no time for science. One or the other had to go, and so I resigned with no regrets. There had once been a day when rounds were a pleasure and filing cabinets were few. Now studysection secretaries and site visitors make decisions that professional peer groups used to control.

Psychiatric chairmen used to be a source of pride to their mentors, but currently, with the unending paperwork demanded of them by federal and state governments and by hospitals, the psychiatric administrator has ceased to be looked upon as a credit to his profession. Some of those who began as investigators assumed the roles of administrators "to help" run large complex institutions. Others have become attorneys and have contributed greatly to the medicolegal problems involving psychiatry. Stone, Watson, and Jonas Rapaport are examples.

Stone states:

> By 1973 American psychiatry at last began to recognize that it was in trouble. But instead of closing ranks to cope with the problems, internecine warfare broke out. There have always been conflicts within psychiatry. The Fifties saw a schism between the dogmatically psychoanalytic and dogmatically organic. During the Sixties, however,

psychiatry moved from these polarities and became a conglomerate. Psychoanalysis lost much of its prestige and authority, and diverse schools of psychotherapy emerged—transactionalists, existentialists, gestaltists, and so forth. The behavior therapists, the sex therapists, the family therapists, and the group therapists all staked out new claims. The behavioristic analysis of mental illness and its treatment became particularly powerful and influential.

The old organically oriented psychiatrists were supplanted by high-powered neuropharmacologists, geneticists, neurobiologists, and neurophysiologists. In this respect, psychiatry for the first time established solid ties with the basic medical sciences. The proliferation of new technology was awesome, but it created such narrow subspecialities within psychiatry that major problems of communication arose not only among those doing different kinds of basic research, but also between the researchers and the clinicians.

Beyond this diversification within the polar positions, there was the blossoming of what can loosely be called social psychiatry. Social psychiatry is in my opinion the other side of the ideological coin 'Psychiatry Kills.' Its claim is that most mental illness can be understood as a manifestation of stress within the social system. Therefore, psychiatry's proper role, if it is to be a preventative discipline, is to deal with factors causing social stress; e.g., racism, sexism, poverty, unemployment, the threat of atomic war, the generation gap. Many of psychiatry's most articulate spokesmen worked in this heady context.

The line between social reform and preventive psychiatry blurred, and enterprising psychiatrists set out to change the world. The problem was that the ambiguity between the goals of social justice and the goals of preventive psychiatry was never clarified. I suppose it never could have been because, at the most profound level, psychiatry —like the rest of medicine—knows something about sickness but almost nothing about the mystery of health. The blueprint is always to eradicate illness, not to create health (Grinker, 1962).

The present conglomerate of psychiatry has been described as having four distinguishable perspectives: social, biological, psychodynamic, and behavioral. Each conceptualizes mental illness—its etiology and its manifestations—in different ways. Such divergent perspectives forced psychiatrists into an uncomfortable choice: either they would strive for a broad eclecticism, condemning themselves to an inevitable superficiality of understanding, or they would dig in, and become isolated in their narrow expertise. In some respects their problems were no different from those confronting the rest of the medical profession, for all physicians face a knowledge explosion; however, psychiatry had still deeper reasons for controversy. Different psychiatrists had fundamentally different conceptions of the nature and extent of the illnesses they treated and now they treated them.

Edward Schwartz, president of the Institute for the Study of Civic Values, wrote (unpublished):

> Recently I was asked to write a grant proposal for a project in Pennsylvania related to adult education. After accepting the offer I discovered that the guidelines for this proposal had to conform to federal specifications. I did endure this remarkable procedure, but shortly thereafter conjured in a horrible nightmare the following letter written to Thomas Jefferson in late July 1776.

July 20, 1776.

Mr. Thomas Jefferson
Continental Congress
Independence Hall
Philadelphia, Pa.

Dear Mr. Jefferson:

We have read your "Declaration of Independence" with great interest. Certainly, it represents a considerable undertaking, and many of your statements do merit serious consideration. Unfortunately, the Declaration as a whole fails to meet recently adopted specifications for proposals to the Crown, so we must return the document to you for further refinement. The questions which follow might assist you in your process of revision.

1. In your opening paragraph you use the phrase "Laws of Nature and Nature's God." What are these laws? In what way are they the criteria on which you base your central arguments? Please document with citations from the recent literature.

2. In the same paragraph you refer to the "opinions of mankind." Whose polling data are you using? Without specific evidence, it seems to us, the "opinions of mankind" are a matter of opinion.

3. You hold certain truths to be "self-evident." Could you please elaborate? If they are as evident as you claim, then it should not be difficult for you to locate the appropriate supporting statistics.

4. "Life, liberty, and the pursuit of Happiness" seem to be the goals of your proposal. These are not measurable goals. If you were to say that "among these is the ability to sustain an average life expectancy in six of the 13 colonies of at least 55 years, and to enable all newspapers in the colonies to print news without outside interference, and to raise the average income of the colonists by 10 percent in the next 10 years," these would be measurable goals. Please clarify.

5. You state that "whenever any Form of Government becomes

destructive of these ends, it is the Right of the People to alter or to abolish it, and to institute a new Government . . . " Have you weighted this assertion against all the alternatives? Or is it predicated solely on the baser instincts?

6. Your description of the existing situation is quite extensive. Such a long list of grievances should precede the statement of goals, not follow it.

7. Your strategy for achieving your goal is not developed at all. You state that the colonies "ought to be Free and Independent States," and that they are "Absolved from All Allegiance to the British Crown." Who or what must change to achieve this objective? In what way must they change? What resistance must you overcome to achieve the change? What specific steps will you take to overcome the resistance? How long will it take? We have found that a little foresight in these areas helps to prevent careless errors later on.

8. Who among the list of signatories will be responsible for implementing your strategy? Who conceived it? Who provided the theoretical research? Who will constitute the advisory committee? Please submit an organizational chart.

9. You must include an evaluation design. We have been requiring this since Queen Anne's War.

10. What impact will your program have? Your failure to include assessment of this inspires little confidence in the long-range prospects of your undertaking.

11. Please submit a PERT diagram, an activity chart, and an itemized budget.

We hope that these comments prove useful in revising your "Declaration of Independence."

Best Wishes,
(Lord North)

The real issue is therapeutic (whether psychological maneuvers can alter genetic destiny). Freud thought so, and so did my father, as a representative of psychotherapists of his day. The real judges of competence is not the external social judges voicing false praises, but one's inner feeling that one has done well.

Fortunately, I devoured the literature in neurology that was so important for my future role as a psychiatric clinician. An area of great concern today is the neurological lesion, its basis for many psychiatric symptoms, which requires depth in neuropsychiatric synthesis and the help of competent clinical psychologists.

Also, at issue today is the need to improve the quality of

psychiatric residents and at least provide a modicum of research personnel, of which there are now too few. Once chosen, the potential investigator can be stimulated and encouraged to engage in appropriate activities. But how do we recruit more of these people? One attempt, which I have described, failed. Actually, I have come to believe that research curiosity and, for that matter, therapeutic skills, although acquired by proper education, rests on some basic preparation. They are either there or they are not.

Another issue of importance is the split between those in practice in the field, clinic, and hospital, and the theoreticians who are ignorant of the practical problems. How else would they still believe that psychiatrists are responsible for primary prevention of mental disease?

Many experienced and competent psychiatrists have experienced an important transition from lack of concern to intense involvement in the psychiatric problems of war. Some, with one excuse or another, managed to stay out and continue their civilian activities. The issue here is what is the psychological difference between those who experienced war and those who did not? Spiegel and I studied our patients and innovated techniques of diagnosis and treatment. We worked hard and learned much of application to later civilian life. The young psychiatrists who were later drafted in peacetime, or during the succeeding years, came for advice and were strongly urged not to sit out the time "bitching," but to read, study, and work for their own improvement, if not for their patients'.

Following World War II, the Group for the Advancement of Psychiatry was organized, and at once, an important issue developed. Dr. Bertram Brown spoke of all of the functions that must engage all psychiatrists, and Dr. Walter Barton emphasized that the primary function of the psychiatrist was to treat the sick as a complete physician—not as a magician or social engineer. This issue still is boiling in psychiatric circles. Where are psychiatrists going, what pathways should they take, and what systems of evaluation should they use? This hot issue already has split psychiatric organizations into political and scientific bodies, to the detriment of progress.

Important issues arose between 1950 and 1965. In all branches of science, so-called basic research received less support. Congress demanded research of *relevance* to the human situation. No one could deny that both basic and applied research in complementary proportions are necessary, but dichotomies now raging as issues are unfortunately primitive ways of thinking.

Without question, psychiatry has extended into obscure areas devoid of control or evaluation, and it is sometimes dangerous. Expressed simply, psychiatry has lost its boundaries. When will we find them again? The *Archives of General Psychiatry,* under my editorship, was an eclectic journal, but it maintained its professional position. Today, under new editorship, the *Archives* has become more concerned with drugs and biochemical processes. As a result, its name, *General Psychiatry,* is no longer appropriate, and it has lost its position as the leading American psychiatric periodical.

One of the crucial issues facing psychiatry today involves diagnosis and classification. It is of the utmost importance to clinical psychiatry and scientific consensus. The need for clinicians and investigators to agree on a combined focus of treatment or research is one of our most crucial priorities. At a time when radical psychiatrists are attempting to sweep the matter away as the "myth of mental illness," we must do our utmost to dispel the notion that diagnosis is unimportant and that only a single patient's problems are what matters. To accept such a limited approach is a retreat from science.

During the last several decades, as we have seen, attempts have been made to incorporate several minor theories in psychiatry into overall unified theory, the most popular of which is general systems theory, which had its foundations in the work of the naturalists of the early part of this century. I have discussed this metatheory at some length because it is valuable both for the clinician and the investigator. An acceptance of its value, however, is greatly at issue, because clinicians fail to grasp its usefulness; psychoanalysts abhor its language; and basic scientists are reluctant to leave their isolated and reductionistic positions.

Another important issue in psychiatry is the nature of the

stress stimuli that end in disease. These cannot merely be assessed quantitatively; what is important is their meaning to the subject.

Anxiety is invariably the first of a sequence of events stimulating defensive or coping devices, whether the stimulus is physical or psychological. But disease is not the only end result; normality may ensue. Strangely, psychiatrists are enmeshed in pathology and have rarely been interested in health or normality, which are not absolutes but are relative to age, society, and culture.

Alexander's specificity hypothesis regarding psychosomatic disturbance is no longer an issue. The term *psychosomatic* is itself a dichotomy. Today, the questions must be framed in a different way: What are the mechanisms by which the mind exerts its influence on the body and vice versa? Investigators are attempting to demonstrate the operation of these mechanisms in specific diseases. Through liaison psychiatry and consultation, they are also attempting to teach nonpsychiatrists how to begin to understand the complex role of the mind in health and disease.

Neurotic disorders are classified by the various overt means by which basic anxiety is defended. Personality disorders have not been studied carefully as to diagnosis and mechanism. Some of the most important issues today are the borderline syndrome and its supposed relationship to schizophrenia and the validity of what are called *narcissistic neuroses.*

The issues involving depressions implicate the question of overwhelming biological source versus psychological factors. Both are essential. Is depression an actual neurosis based on faulty cerebral biochemistry, or is it a dynamic process precipitated by life events? I think it is a cycle precipitated at any arc by a wide variety of stimuli; once started, it tends to take the identical form and last until its natural decline.

The issues concerning therapy are both professional and legalistic. The wide variety of treatments now employed makes it essential that we provide for evaluation of results by means of follow-up studies over a lengthy period of time. There are no hard data that can evaluate the real results, and there may never be any. To quantify the relative success of various psychotherapies, pharmacotherapies, and group, family, and encounter groups is virtually impossible. What are the common factors in the end result? How important are faith and the subjective transactions in the therapeutic alliance of therapist and patient or are there objective scientific criteria not yet discovered?

Who is to be educated and how, is dependent on the question "for what?" Fundamentally, all professional education should turn out competent general psychiatrists who may then specialize in one or another special functions, such as research, therapy of some peer groups, and teaching. Medical students should receive an opportunity to know enough to make sensible choices. At least, they should be taught the elements of psychosomatic factors.

Peer groups currently are separated for study and treatment, as the life cycle is being viewed as a succession of stages with separate problems and susceptibilities requiring special therapeutic procedures.

Investigators in the field of clinical psychiatry are not numerous, but there are many concerned with parts of the total field, from genetics to sociology. The clinical researcher, whose task consists of developing organizational principles and discovering the processes of control and regulation necessary to maintain integration and prevent disorganization and regression, has not functioned effectively. Too much time is spent in developing little pieces of information, and there is not enough concern with larger issues. The time has arrived to "think big," which I have tried to do.

Psychosocial factors are currently important issues influencing health, health services, and community well-being. They stem from the psychology of the individual as it relates to the structure and function of social groups. They include social characteristics, such as patterns of interaction within kinship or occupation groups; cultural characteristics, such as traditional ways of solving conflict; and psychological characteristics, such as attitudes, beliefs, and personality factors.

These factors are interdependent, and the way in which they affect the healthy development and functioning of individuals cannot be understood without considering the more global aspects of society—the organization and division of work; the institutions and structures forming the sociopolitical systems; the values, norms, and codes regulating the behavior of individuals and groups; and the cultural heritage.

All sciences, including their primitive precursor, mythology, are closely involved in their contemporary social matrix, either directly or indirectly. Psychiatry is in part a social science, since man is a social animal and his individuality is only approximate, not ultimate. Society demands, requests, condones, and condemns some forms of psychiatry, just as it deals with other intellectual trends in its component members or groups. In this sense, psychiatry is *in* society. In another sense, psychiatry and society are two systems closely related to each other by way of transactions between their interfaces. To understand this relationship, one has to designate those parts of society with which psychiatry exchanges information. These include the family, neighborhood and other geographical partitions, school, police, church, and work, etc.

Society defines mental health for its population. In answer to his teacher's question in Mell's cartoon, "Ira, don't you want to be known as a normal, average, American boy?" Ira answered, "No, I want to be like all the others." Health is a value system dependent on the place, time, and population. Each set of conditions imposes a threshold beyond which deviance becomes intolerable and is termed illness. Anselm Strauss (1964) has stated that we need much more sophistication about normality—a sociological range and differentiation of normal behavior is now almost altogether missing in psychiatrists' thinking. Society not only lays down standards of health and also the acceptance of the secondary role of illness, but also the means by which coping mechanisms may be used in the stresses of development, which seem to be phase-specific, and the threatening events and crises in our turbulent lives. Normality and illness are only polarities of a wide range of integrations—when strained, the organismic systems respond according to the processes by which the many subvariances have become integrated—thus, the degree of health and illness in the stress responses reveals the quality of and quantifies the integration.

Our concepts of the multiple causes of emotional and cognitive disturbances and their treatment are certainly dependent on our view as observers of the transactions between social, personality, and cultural processes. Granted the innate biological basis of some diseases, are subsequent personality deviances due to difficult or traumatic experiences in early family life? To what degree do conflicts in society contribute to psychological malfunctioning? We have begun to realize that phases of the life cycle involve different social problems: We divide the life span into several phases of childhood, adolescence, young adulthood, adulthood, and aging. Each has its own conflicts, predispositions, susceptibilities, forms of deviance, and applicable therapies.

Society is not a uniform process. Ours is not a unitary society, as the mythology of a melting pot indicated. Indeed, it is a pluralistic society composed of various ethnic, socioeconomic, and racial groups. Our states and regions are still differentiated by their geography, resources, and industries.

Just as we cannot speak of *a* psychiatry, we cannot speak of *a* society. Where a person is born and where he lives, is educated, and works exposes him to different societies and cultures that make demands on him and to which he must adapt. Moving from one place to another even so short a distance from a city to its suburbs or adapting to the destruction of a neighborhood to build a throughway requires some form of coping.

Thus, infinite systems are always in constant movement, with individuals growing, maturing, and developing into different phases of the life cycle; society is changing with incredible speed due to technological discoveries. A one-to-one relationship, a matching between personality or psychopathy and sociocultural factors, is thus difficult. This has always been so, although psychiatrists have ignored the rapidly shifting internal and external factors involved in psychiatry. Recognition now results in less certainty, despite greater sophistication in research, as the possibility of controlling many variables has become more difficult.

There is a more pressing ethical issue for the psychiatrist than that of keeping the mentally retarded and the hopelessly senile alive. With increasing confidence that there is a biological basis to the development of the schizophrenic system, we should be aware that we are increasing the genetic pool by the use of anti-schizophrenic drugs that enable us to discharge from warehouses patients who are thereby free to marry and bear children.

I am not sanguine about the future—not only because we are in an era of anti-intellectualism, which includes antipsychiatric attitudes, but, most important, because I see the psychiatric profession itself downgraded by destructive and splintering behavior within its own ranks.

The role that our society has imposed on us is a staggering—and a frightening—one. On February 5, 1963, former President John F. Kennedy, in a message to the Eighty-eighth Congress, clearly identified the national issue of the problem of mental illness and the need for returning mental illness to the mainstream of American medicine and for upgrading mental health services. On October 31, 1963, the Community Mental Health Act was passed, mandating the National Institute of Mental Health to establish and fund community mental health centers, each to be located in a homogeneous catchment area of about 75,000 to 200,000 people and to encompass several essential services, with additional optional ones. Historically, this event represented the culmination of the effort to view mental health and mental illness as a national responsibility, a view that had been initiated in the mid-nineteenth century.

Much later, the courts ruled that mentally ill and mentally retarded patients had the right to adequate care and treatment, which was not universally available because of insufficient personnel and funds. Our professional societies have endorsed this right, although the definition of what is adequate is still lacking, and enforcement of this ruling is difficult. Psychiatrists seem to be seduced by every new form of treatment, "Riding madly," as I have said, "in all directions."

The legalities recently developed have resulted in a war between psychiatrists and their enemies—nonpsychiatric physicians, lawyers, judges, and social scientists. Psychiatrists have been accused of killing, even by civil libertarians.

Andrew Watson spoke of the rights of the mentally ill and the diminished responsibility of criminals. I confronted both of these issues when I testified in both the Heirens and the Speck cases. The McNaughen ruling of 1843 was a good deal simpler. It merely demanded that the accused be capable of discriminating between right and wrong.

Though the Durham rule stated by Judge Bazelon depended on psychiatric diagnoses of mental disease or defect, it too was unsatisfactory. We have also been catapulted into other legal issues–including juvenile delinquency, battered children, involuntary hospitalization, adoption, divorce, informed consent, and malpractice, etc. Our psychiatric hospitals and societies are less busy with their professional activities than with their defensive posture against many recent ill-advised laws.

The new mental health codes (one is in Illinois) require much more study because they are being formulated by lawyers rather than psychiatrists. In fact, psychiatrists are forming unions to fight the government's attempts to control bargaining fees, type of treatment, and time allotted for treatment and results, using false normals. The doctor-patient relationship is being radically altered, and the doctor is no longer an independent contractor but an employee.

The federal bureaucracy and its multiple and changing regulations have converted the scientific hero into a villain in our society. Furthermore, the local medical schools and teaching and research hospitals have had to create their own bureaucracies to match those of the federal government, often without understanding the language of the multiple regulations.

Scientific research must be recognized for what it is, a social rather than a business activity, even though it generates the same outward patterns of growth. First, informal cooperation becomes organized; then, the organization eventually becomes laden down by a bureaucracy in which originality of thought at the expense of routine efficiency is discouraged. A working consensus between the research scientist and his legislative and regulatory counterparts can only be achieved by a dialogue that includes a rational analysis of alternatives. With the installation of a new national administration, a fresh opportunity exists for the scientific community to initiate this dialogue with government for the benefit of all concerned.

Without discussing bureaucracy in detail, Ruesch (1975) reiterates that the goal of bureaucracy is to ensure an impartial administration of office. However, inasmuch as the psychiatrist's task is not related to public office but to the individual, the acceptance of bureaucratic practices undermines his activities. Exposure to bureaucracy begins with the resident's contact with the training center, which to a large measure is supported by the government; for his medical and postdoctoral education, such a trainee frequently receives stipends administered by a government agency, foundation, or the like. It is in this institutional and subsidized environment that the young psychiatrist spends his formative years. While the organizational shell of the institution of which he is a part reflects the impersonal technological social order, the clinical teachers emphasize individual development, self-realization, and personal relations. It is understandable that the young doctor is confused by the contradictions.

The conflict between the psychiatrist as an individual doctor and as a member of the total social group brings into focus the principle of the part in relation to the whole. In the biological field, stress applied to the organism may strain one or more parts, intensifying activity, but often leading to disintegration. If the disintegration is not irreversible, the total organism has the capacity for reorganization. In the field of social sciences, the problem of stress as it strains the social group is well known. The effect on the individual may often be *disintegration,* another term for personal sickness. The individual as a component of a social order has limited resistance to stress and cannot be substituted by an auxiliary organ or system. He will succumb unless removed from the social group for special care or unless the stress that has impinged upon him is terminated. Mankind has developed social institutions that are based upon the principle of individual dignity and protect or revive the sick person who has succumbed to social stresses.

In our present-day concept of health and disease, we recognize no sharp separation, but only a continuum. Furthermore, we see no essential difference in etiology between somatic and psychological disease. Today, we know that somatic disease is more than the result of an accidental invasion by a demoniacal bacterium but requires a susceptibility based on the state of the whole organism, including its emotional stability. Likewise, those who become psychologically sick are reacting to more than current life situations, but are prepared by earlier experiences in the family or other social groups to succumb with greater or lesser ease to specific stresses. In fact, an individual's value system, ethics, ideals, and conscience are the result of past social experiences. Both those past and present precipitating life situations are the result of transactions between the individual and the society in which he lives.

Society, which is thus partly the cause of an individual's difficulties, has always looked for protection against what it has caused. It isolates the physically contagious in special hospitals. It incarcerates the criminal in jails. It institutionalizes the psychotic in mental hospitals. In preliterate societies, the individuals reacting psychologically to stress to become deviants could migrate to less stressful or more suitable social groups. In the Middle Ages, the weary and oppressed found sanctuary in the Church. Today, those who cannot be tolerated within a social group because of their threat to the social order can be given no sanctuary which is not at the same time a safeguard against them. Hospitals and doctors are required, prisoners need rehabilitation and sensible parole opportunities, and the psychotic requires adequate institutional housing and therapy.

What about the individual who is not sick enough for isolation? Today, he finds sanctuary and treatment only in the doctor's office or in the special modern psychiatric hospital. To be helped, he must tell all his problems, his deepest secrets, his most intimate interpersonal relations, and all future asocial acts. Furthermore, confessions made to a psychiatrist and reported would probably have no validity in court, since they only constitute hearsay evidence. Perhaps the psychiatrist should be required to report projected or intended asocial deeds. The psychiatrist is always aware of the danger that his patient may not be able to control his feelings and limit them to fantasy or verbalizations. He is constantly aware of the danger that the patient may act out his impulses. If the psychiatrist sees that the patient may act out an aggressive or asocial impulse, he is the first to initiate a restraining influence as a representative of society, demanding incarceration or hospitalization, thereby preventing suicide or homicide. The psychiatrist can recognize these tendencies when others cannot. No judge can decide these facts.

Medicine has operated for many centuries under the Oath of Hippocrates, the common law of medicine, which states that patient-doctor communications are privileged and that these must not be divulged unless permitted by the patient. During the age of Hippocrates and the enlightened Greek school of medicine, there were no psychiatrists. Today, psychiatry, as a special field of medicine concerned with treatment of the individual's needs in a complex and ever more stressful social order, is growing in geometric proportions. Today, the psychiatrist more than anyone else is the professional person who protects the dignity and rights of the individual sufferer.

The common law, as understood by the legal profession, is constantly adapted to changes in the social structure and is modified to fit contemporary problems. This common law should now take cognizance of the special close patient-doctor relationship in the psychiatrist's role of treatment of the sick individual, of his role with workers in industry, in his counseling capacity, and in his function in marital clinics. In all these, secrets relating to family, employer, and larger social groups must not be divulged.

I believe that the solution to what has become an endless and sometimes bitter verbal controversy between psychiatrists and psychologists, with threats and lawsuits, is not a manifestation of a revolutionary change, but rather evidence of evolutionary experimentation. All professionals in mental health disciplines—psychiatrists, psychologists, social workers, and nurses—should be cooperatively involved in the process of providing care through overlapping functions.

As the twentieth century is nearing its close, many people are asking questions about the future. In fact, all sciences are looking ahead to determine how their disciplines will fare in the century ahead, by means of conferences, symposia, and a new science called *futurology*. Psychiatrists are probably more concerned about the future, because their present is, to say the least, disquieting. We are engulfed by scientism, general feelings of frustration and futility as American political and economic conditions are changing radically for the worse. Unfortunately, the public has little patience, and its demands for crash programs and immediate gains have been expressed by bureaucrats who advocate support of only "mission-oriented" research. The community mental health wave promised primary prevention of mental illness, which is far off in the future. Perhaps it is unattainable because of the continuing conflict between man's drives as an evolved animal and his socialized and social controls.

The emphasis on the quantity and equality of treatment for all has prematurely sacrificed the individuality of persons in trouble and has seriously weakened sound scientific investigations. New antischizophrenic, antidepressive, and antimanic drugs have been widely misused for relief of almost any psychological complaint, just as the "miracle drugs" are demanded for conditions for which they are ineffective. These psychotropic drugs have and will continue to advance our knowledge of the biochemical constituents of cerebral activities as a part of the functional analysis of disorders involved in psychiatric diseases.

The future of psychiatry hinges on changes in the shifting behaviors of man in a changing society that we cannot predict at this time. Shifts in family constellations are reflected in increased urbanization, changes in the kinds of parenting, and other social and economic factors, which may result in changes in the kinds of coping available to succeeding generations.

As psychiatrists, we cannot reorganize society, we are novices in politics, and we have not yet caught up with the explosive progress in biological psychiatry to develop a modern neuropsychiatry. As Arthur (1973) states,

> Social psychiatry, which includes the study of the impingement of social phenomena upon the genesis, manifestations, and treatment of mental and physical illness, has in recent decades an increasingly im-

> portant part of psychiatry. The epidemiology and taxonomy of mental illness, social factors in the onset and course of disease, transcultural psychiatry, the hospital viewed in social terms, and community psychiatry are all fields that have shown great expansion. But the results of the experiences of community psychiatry and of social psychiatric studies have played a major role in the development of a crisis of identity within the professional activities for a psychiatrist are currently in dispute.

All of this means that psychiatry is necessarily part of the process of change. It reinforces the idea that solid, well-programmed research in all disciplines of psychiatry should be supported and greatly extended if our civilization does not nurture the seeds of its own destruction. We no longer can afford the luxury of making public generalization for narcissistic purposes.

The future rests on establishing sound and dedicated goals and methods for the educational process. Unfortunately, there are many obstacles, many outside pressures over which we have limited control. Our most crucial task, let me repeat, is to get the student to recognize that there are no dichotomies between genetics and environment and no sharp differentiations between levels of development and phases of the life cycle. To understand that is to accept a philosophy of ontology in relation to scientific disciplines and to the therapeutic aspects of medicine (Grinker, 1971).

Such an understanding, I believe, must point toward a new direction for a curriculum of education that is multidisciplinary and not entirely medical. Some of it should be incorporated in the university and some in the premedical years. In any event, it must be seen as a continuous process. The goals are to give to the student a concept of the totality of the life cycle, the transactional relationship among its parts, the components of these parts, and to avoid reductionism on the one hand and a distorted humanism on the other. If we could augment this picture with contributions from other scientific disciplines and from each of the applied medical sciences, then, even with a variety of approaches and differences in methods, a concept of all of life would emerge, including its so-called healthy and sick components. Then we would have true unitary thinking.

In my long professional career, I have had the good fortune to live in an exciting professional era. It began in the 1920s nourished by the illusory promise of the mental hygiene movement: "Do as we tell you, and mental illness will be abolished." Unfortunately, the promise was not accompanied by a prescription as to how and when. Then, slowly, psychoanalysis permeated American psychiatry, changing it from a sterile diagnostic exercise into a dynamic explanatory understanding of unconscious motivation, conflict, defense, and compulsion to repeat eternally inadequate learning or neurotic solutions. This influence reached its height after World War II. At the same time it seemed to the Chicago group, led by Alexander, that chronic physical diseases could be caused in part by specific repressed emotions, and that short-term therapy, by uncovering or exposing these, could alleviate the specific symptoms.

Again, psychiatry was oversold. In addition to insufficient manpower, psychoanalysis (theoretically fascinating though it is) did not cure. The specificity hypothesis did not hold against contrary evidence, and so we returned to the laboratory to study stress responses and psychophysiological relations by experimenting on animals, as well as observing humans. Optimism seemed to have disappeared because it was built on faith in dramatic breakthroughs. The result, however was really salutary, because psychiatry entered a new era. From a medical specialty with concerns limited to diagnosis and treatment, it became a scientific field comprising many parts, from genetics to sociology and anthropology—a general system.

Then, several advances were made. The first was the introduction of new drugs to alleviate psychoses: schizophrenia, then depressions, and recently, mania. All these plus a widening range of psychological therapies for individuals, couples, families, and groups, give hope to many. Most state hospitals are no longer snakepits, and people are discharged to their home before they can become career patients. In addition, the drugs stimulated intense research on the biochemistry of the nervous system and on systems of transmission of various elements in the causal chains of function.

Finally, community mental health programs have been developing to deliver care to the indigent within their own environments. Use is being made of community resources instead of hospitals, and crisis intervention for people in trouble is available for the many. We are expanding the vista of psychiatry as a right, like any health care system, available to all, not just those who can buy interminable treatment for minor discomforts.

Naturally, there are many legitimate arguments about what is most important, how to train the general psychiatrist effectively, and on what the tax dollars should be concentrated. Ideologies are in conflict, but the current chaotic state is at least exciting and promises that, with proper systems of control and evaluation, we will eventually know what is best for whom and even perhaps how to prevent some forms of mental illness or social incompetence.

Regrettably, however, these new and exciting changes have recently slowed down. Funds from governmental agencies and private philanthropy have entered a period of drought, and many research, training, and service functions have had to be curtailed or abandoned because billions of dollars are being wasted each year on military expenditures. Policy within our current federal administration is more oriented to punishment for deviance than to determining causes, especially of drug dependency and abuse and juvenile delinquency.

But even in the face of these frustrations, I shall, in my remaining years, as I always have, continue to promote the best possible care for patients in hospital and community clinics, to facilitate the research of others, as well as containing my own, and to extend the teaching program at all levels. I plan this all with a degree of optimism that existing obstacles, as well as those inevitably arising in the future, will be met. As we teach small children, "Obstacles are what need to be overcome." Although there are relatively few physical obstacles that man's technology cannot overcome, the same cannot as yet be said about our major obstacle against human progress, man himself. We are currently observing in all walks of life decreasing standards and levels of integrity, decreasing controls of hostility, and, in defense, a generalized increase in paranoid attitudes.

No one can doubt that all is not well in our expanding society, even though not one of the defects that is pinpointed by a specific name is a new problem. All have existed for decades, even centuries, as characteristics of civilizations that spawn major urban concentrations, which in turn tend to destroy the civilizations in which they develop. Under these circumstances, the balance between personal and community life vacillates and often becomes precarious (Langer, 1964).

Whether we call these changes *revolution,* although this word has come to mean almost any kind of dissent, or *evolution,* our perception is a matter of the speed of the change. In revolution, change is rapid and seems to constitute, or is interpreted as, a crisis. In evolution, it is much slower and often imperceptible, except in retrospect. Most violent revolutions, with the major exception of the American Revolution, have espoused the goals of freedom, but have been followed by periods of tyranny. Evolutions, whether biological or social, are often regressive, and the mutations are frequently lethal. Whether the end result is progress is a value judgment better left to posterity.

I do not believe that what we are witnessing is a revolution, nor the beginnings of one. There does not seem to be a threat to our established system of government, although certainly we have seen a good many focal confrontations during the past two decades. Various explanations for this unrest have been offered as causes by persons whose professions lead them to specific biases. The psychologist talks about student paranoia; the sociologist about a characteristically violent American society—or conflict between haves and have nots; the psychiatrist about racist and generational hate and guilt. But these observations are derived from frames of reference too close to the behaviors and too narrow for inclusive generalities.

I believe that we are witnessing at all levels of our social network a conflict based on dualistic thinking, the polarities of which are personal or individual freedom as against social structures maintaining the functions of regulation and control. Each has moved speedily and quantitatively to become antagonists to the other. The greater the demand for freedom, the more repressive the measures set into action. The more restrictive the controls to dampen freedoms, the more protest and violence. With this frame of reference, no single cause can be accepted; instead a general approach to all of life, whether biological, psychological, or social, is more adequate. Paul Weiss (1973), in discussing organization from cell to culture, epitomized this approach: "I mean the operation of a principle of order that stabilizes and preserves the total pattern of the group activity of a huge mass of semi-autonomous elements."

With rigid order, we have tyranny; with no order, anarchy. What we need is "order in the gross and freedom in the small," a unitary form of thinking toward which man has been evolving for centuries. True, it is difficult to maintain such a view of life in the midst of stress and its evoked emotional responses. Those who need the myth of single causes and promises of supernatural solutions find it especially difficult to accept this kind of thinking.

Currently we are witnessing back-and-forth swings in control and expression that differ from those of previous decades only in the rapidity and the range of the shifts of emphasis. The emotionality of commitment often results in the destruction of the protestor's own environment: black's housing, students' school buildings, or an organization's principles. On the other hand, the emotionality of the regulators of orders results in gassing, shooting, and severe prison sentences. Reason always fails, temporarily, before the onslaught of mass irrationality.

We must continue to search for new experiences, for dreams of a better world focused on other than excessive material advantages; experiences that transcend homeostatic and sociostatic traditionally set goals. Goal-changing thinking and behavior are radical only in their form, not because of their innovation contents. They are truly the hopes for progress.

It seems that I have covered the future of psychiatry as defined both from a medical and scientific point of view with broad sweeps of the brush. It is impossible for any one department or institute to cover the entire ground. We are greatly dependent upon the component sciences that make up the whole field of psychiatry. The problem with which we must deal, is what aspects of the various sciences, what contributions, or indeed, what individuals within these sciences contribute something in the near future. It may be that we are entirely dependent upon chance opportunities of getting specific representatives of scientific disciplines to work in a psychiatric department or institute.

In my lifetime of work in the field of psychiatry, I have been exposed to and part of the changing cycles: from the low point of overemphasis on the medical model, to the high point of psychodynamic dominance, to the current conglomeration devoid of a rational system, with every mental health discipline involved in conflicts over authority and power. We can only hope that the golden era of the midcentury (Grinker, 1953a) will someday return, at least in part.

REFERENCES

Abraham, K.: *Selected Papers on Psychoanalysis.* New York, Basic, 1960.

Alexander, F.: *Psychosomatic Medicine.* New York, Norton, 1950.

———: *The Scope of Psychoanalysis, 1921-1961.* New York, Basic, 1961.

Alexander, F., French, T.M., and Pollock, G.H.: *Psychosomatic Specificity.* U of Chicago Pr, 1968, vol. 1.

Alexander, F. and Selesnick, T.: *The History of Psychiatry.* New York, Har-Row, 1966.

Anthony, E.J.: Research as an academic function of child psychiatry. *Arch Gen Psychiatry, 21*:385-391, 1969.

Apter, N.S.: Alternative of ego functions in chronic schizophrenia. *Arch Gen Psychiatry, 1*:622, 1959.

Arieti, S.: *Interpretation of Schizophrenia.* New York, Brunner-Mazel, 1955.

———: The present status of psychiatry theories. *Am J Psychiatry, 124*:619-629, 1968.

———: *Creativity: The Magic Synthesis.* New York, Basic, 1976.

Arthur, R.J.: *Social Psychiatry: An Overview.* Navy Medical Neuropsychiatric Research Report no. 73-74. Washington, D.C., U.S. Govt Print. Office, 1973.

Ashby, W.R.: *Design for a Brain.* New York, Wiley, 1965.

Bailey, P.: *Sigmund the Unserene.* Springfield, Thomas, 1965.

Basowitz, H., Persky, H., Korchin, S., and Grinker, R.R., Sr.: *Anxiety and Stress.* New York, Blakiston, 1955.

Bateson, G.: *Steps to an Ecology of Mind.* San Francisco, Chandler, 1972.

Beck, S.J.: *Psychological Processes in the Schizophrenic Adaptation.* New York, Grune, 1965.

Beck, T.: *Depression.* New York, Har-Row, 1967.

Becker, C.: *Everyman His Own Historian: Essays on History and Politics.* New York, Appleton-Century-Crofts, 1935.

Bender, L.: Twenty years of clinical research on schizophrenia. *J Autism Child Schizo, 1*:115-118, 1971.

Bender, L. and Freedman, M.A.: A study of the first three years in the maturation of schizophrenic children. *Q J Child Behav, 4*:245-271, 1952.

Benedek, T.: *Studies in Psychosomatic Medicine.* New York, Ronald, 1952.

———: Toward the biology of a depressive constellation. *J Am Psychoanal Assoc, 4*:389-402, 1956.

Bertalanffy, L. von: Mind and body re-examined. *J Hum Psychol, 6*:113-138, 1966.

———: General theory of systems: Application of psychology. *Soc Sci Info, 6*:125-136, 1967.

———: *General Systems Theory*. New York, Braziller, 1968.

Bibring, E.: *The Mechanism of Depression*. New York, Intl Univs Pr, 1953.

Bleuler, E.: *Dementia Praecox or the Group of Schizophrenics*. Translated by J. Zinkin. New York, Intl Univs Pr, 1950.

Bleuler, M.: Conception of schizophrenia within the last fifty years and today. *Proc R Soc Med, 56*:945-952, 1963. Reviewed by A. Lewis in *Psychol Med, 3*:385-392, 1973.

———: The long-term course of the schizophrenic psychosis. *Psychol Med, 4*:224-254, 1974.

Boring, E.G. and Lindsey, G. (Eds.): *A History of Psychology in Autobiography*. New York, Meredith Corp, 1967, vol. 5.

Bowlby, J.: *Attachment and Loss*. New York, Basic, 1969, vol. 1.

Bozzetti, L.P. and MacMurray, J.P.: Contemporary concepts of aging. *Psychiatr Ann, 7*:117-127, 1977.

Bronowski, J.: *The Philosophy of Karl P. Popper*. The Hague, The Netherlands, Library of Living Philosophers, Mouton. Humanities, 1974.

Brueke, C. von: Quoted in Cannon, W.: *The Way of an Investigator: A Scientist's Experience in Medical Research*. New York, Norton, 1945.

Bry, I. and Rifkin, A.: Freud and the history of ideas. *Mental Health Review Index*. New York, Bry and Rifkin, 1962.

Campbell, M.C.: *Destiny and Disease*. New York, Norton, 1935.

Cannon, W.: *Wisdom of the Body*. New York, Norton, 1963.

Caplan, G.: *An Approach to Community Mental Health*. New York, Grune, 1961.

Carpenter, W.T., Barthos, J., Strauss, J., and Hank, A.: Signs and symptoms as predictors of outcome: A report on the international pilot study of schizophrenia. *Am J Psychiatry, 135*:940-945, 1978.

Cavanaugh, J., Jr.: Psychopolitics. *Curr Concepts Psychiatry*, Mar.-Apr., 1978.

Childs, C.M.: *Patterns and Problems of Development*. U of Chicago Pr, 1941.

Coehlio, G.U., Hamburg, D.A., and Adams, J.E. (Eds.): *Coping and Adaptation*. New York, Basic, 1974.

Coggseshall, L.T. (Ed.): *Planning for Medical Progress through Education*. Report submitted to the Association of American Medical Colleges, Evanston, Illinois, 1965.

Coghill, G.E.: *Anatomy and the Problem of Behavior*. London, Cambridge U Pr, 1929.

Deutsch, A.: *The Story of GAP*. Brochure. New York, GAP, 1959.

Dunbar, H.F.: *Emotions and Bodily Changes*. New York, Columbia U Pr, 1935.

Dunham, H.W.: Sociocultural studies of schizophrenia. *Arch Gen Psychiatry, 24*:201-214, 1971.

Eissler, K.R.: *Medical Orthodoxy and the Future of Psychoanalysis.* New York, Intl Univs Pr, 1965.

Emerson, A.E.: Dynamic homeostasis: A unifying principle in organic, social, ethical evolution. *Sci Monthly, 78*:67-85, 1954.

Engel, G.: The need for a new medical model: A challenge for biological science. *Science, 196*:128-196, 1971.

Erikson, E.H.: Identity and the life cycle. *Psychol Issues, 1*:1-71, 1959.

Escalona, S. and Herder, S.M.: *Prediction and Outcome.* New York, Basic, 1959; Chicago, Aldine, 1968.

Fraiberg, S., Adelson, W., and Shapiro, U.: Ghosts in the nursery. *J Am Acad Child Psychiatry, 14*:387-421, 1975.

Frank, J.D.: The two faces of psychiatry. *J Nerv Ment Dis, 164*:3-7, 1977.

Frenkel-Brunswick, E.: *Psychoanalysis and the Unity of Science.* Proceedings of the Academy of Arts and Science, New York, 1952.

Freud, A.: *Difficulties in the Path of Psychoanalysis.* New York, Intl Univs Pr, 1957.

——: *Diagnostic Skills and Their Truth in Psychoanalysis.* London, Hogarth, 1976.

Freud, S.: Mourning and melancholia. *The Collected Papers of Sigmund Freud.* London, Hogarth, 1917, vol. 4.

Fromm-Reichman, F.: *Principles of Intensive Psychotherapy.* U of Chicago Pr, 1950.

Garber, B.: *Follow-up of Hospitalized Adolescents.* New York, Brunner-Mazel, 1972.

Gardner, R.W.: Organismic equilibration and the energy-structure quality in psychoanalytic theory: An attempt at theoretical refinement. *J Am Psychonal Assoc, 17*:3-41, 1969.

Garmezy, N.: Process and reactive schizophrenia. In Jackson, D.D. (Ed.): *The Etiology of Schizophrenia.* New York, Basic, 1960.

Gedo, J.E.: Studies on hysteria. *J Am Psychoanal Assoc, 12*:734-751, 1964.

Gerard, R.W. and Grinker, R.R., Sr.: Regenerative possibilities of the central nervous system. *Arch Neurol Psychiatry, 26*:469-484, 1931.

Giannitrapani, D.: Schizophrenia in EEG spectral analysis. *Electromyogr EEG Clin Neurophysiol, 36*:377-386, 1974.

Gill, M.M. and Holzman, P. (Eds.): *Psychology versus Metapsychology: Psychoanalytic Essays in Memory of George S. Klein.* New York, Psychological Bulletin, 1976.

Gitelson, M.: Communication from the president about neopsychoanalytic movement. *Arch Gen Psychiatry, 12*:113-125, 1965.

Glover, E.: *On the Early Development of the Mind.* London, Harcourt, Brace and Co., 1933.

Goldstein, D.: *The Organism: A Holistic Approach to Biology.* New York, Am Bk Co, 1939.

Graham, W.F. and Graham, D.T.: Relationship of specific attitudes and emotions to certain bodily diseases. *Psychosom Med, 14*:243-251, 1952.

Graubard, S.R. (Ed.): American higher education: Toward an uncertain future. Preface. *Daedalus, 1*:ix, 1974.
Grinker, R.R., Jr.: Ego, insight and will-power. *Arch Gen Psychiatry, 5*: 91-102, 1961a.
———: Imposture as a form of mastery. *Arch Gen Psychiatry, 5*:449-452, 1961b.
———: Self-esteem and adaptation. *Arch Gen Psychiatry, 9*:414-415, 1963.
———: Complementary psychotherapy: Treatment of "associated" pairs. *Am J Psychiatry, 123*:633-638, 1966.
Grinker, R.R., Sr.: Parkinsonism following carbon monoxide poisoning. *J Nerv Ment Dis, 64*:17, 1926.
———: Hypothalamic functions in psychosomatic interrelations. *Psychosom Med, 1*:19, 1939.
———: Sigmund Freud: A few reminiscences of a personal contact. *J Orthopsychiatry, 10*:850, 1940.
———: Electroencephalographic studies of corticohypothalamic relations in schizophrenia. *Am J Psychiatry, 98(3)*:385-392, 1941a.
———: Neurosurgical treatment of certain abnormal mental states. Panel discussion. *JAMA, 117*:517-527, 1941b.
———: Narcosynthesis. *Psychoanalytic Therapy.* New York, Ronald, 1946.
——— (Ed.): *Mid-Century Psychiatry.* Springfield, Thomas, 1953a.
———: *Psychosomatic Research.* New York, Norton, 1953b; Aronson, 1973.
———: Introduction. In Beck, S.J. (Ed): *The Six Schizophrenias.* Research Monograph no. 6. New York, Am Orthopsychiatric Assoc, 1954.
———: The Institute for Psychosomatic and Psychiatric Research and Training. *Mental Hospitals.* Washington, D.C., APA, 1956a.
———: *Toward a Unified Theory of Human Behavior.* New York, Basic, 1956b.
———: A transactional model for psychotherapy. *Arch Gen Psychiatry, 1*:1, 1959.
———: "Mentally healthy" young males (homoclites). *Arch Gen Psychiatry, 6*:405, 1962.
———: A psychoanalytic historical island in Chicago (1911-12). *Arch Gen Psychiatry, 8*:392, 1963a.
———: A dynamic story of the "homoclite." In Masserman, J.M. (Ed.): *Science and Psychoanalysis.* New York, Grune, 1963b, vol. 6.
———: Psychiatry rides madly in all directions. *Arch Gen Psychiatry, 10*: 228, 1964a.
———: A struggle for eclecticism. *Am J Psychiatry, 121*:451, 1964b.
———: Research potential of departments of psychiatry in general hospitals. In Kaufman, M.R. (Ed.): *The Psychiatric Unit in a General Hospital.* New York, Intl Univs Pr, 1965a.
———: The sciences of psychiatry: Fields, fences, and riders. *Am J Psychiatry, 122*:367, 1965b.
———: "Open-system" psychiatry. *Am J Psychoanal, 26*:115, 1966a.

———: The specificity of response to stress stimuli. *Arch Gen Psychiatry, 14*:624, 1966b.

———: *Toward a Unified Theory of Human Behavior,* 2nd ed. New York, Basic, 1967.

———: The phenomena of depressions. In Katz, M.M., Cole, J.O., and Barton, W.E. (Eds.): *The Roles and Methodology of Classification in Psychiatry and Psychopathology.* Chevy Chase, Maryland, U.S. Dept. of Health, Education and Welfare, Public Health Service, 1968.

———: An essay on schizophrenia and science. *Arch Gen Psychiatry, 20*:1-25, 1969a.

———: Psychiatry in our dangerous world. In Heseltine, G.F.D. (Ed.): *Psychiatric Research in Our Changing World.* Amsterdam, The Netherlands, Excerpts Medica Foundation, 1969b.

———: The continuing search for meaning. *Am J Psychiatry, 127*:725-731, 1970a.

———: Foreword. In Hamburg, D.A. (Ed.): *Psychiatry as a Behavioral Science.* Englewood Cliffs, New Jersey, P-H, 1970b.

———: Biomedical education as a system. *Arch Gen Psychiatry, 24*:291-298, 1971.

———: Changing styles in psychoses and borderline states. *Am J Psychiatry, 130*:151-152, 1973.

———: Anhedonia and depression. In Anthony, E.J. and Benedek, T. (Eds.): *Depression and Human Existence.* Boston, Little, 1975a.

———: De la alienación a la adaptación. *El Cansan Cio de la Vida,* Madrid, 1975b.

———: Dichotomies, states, and structures. *Am J Psychiatry, 132*:739-740, 1975c.

———: *Psychiatry in Broad Perspective.* New York, Behavioral Pubns, 1975d.

———: Reminiscences of Dr. Roy R. Grinker. *J Acad Psychoanal, 3*:211-233, 1975e.

———: The role of psychiatry in society. In Kriegman, G. et al. (Eds.): *American Psychiatry: Past, Present, and Future.* Charlotteville, U of Va Pr, 1975f.

———: Many concepts, no grand theory, and sparse data. *Contemp Psychol, 21*:38-40, 1976.

———: Borderline syndrome: Phenomenological view. In Harticollis, P. (Ed): *Borderline Personality Disorders.* New York, Intl Univs Pr, 1977.

Grinker, R.R., Sr., Goldstein, I., Heath, R., Oken, D., and Shipman, W.: Study in psychophysiology of muscle tension. I. Response specificity. *Arch Gen Psychiatry, 11*:322, 1964.

Grinker, R.R., Sr., Hamburg, D.A., Sabshin, M., Board, F., Korchin, S., Basowitz, H., Heath, R., and Persky, H.: Classification and rating of emotional experiences. *Arch Neurol Psychiatry, 79*:415, 1958.

Grinker, R.R., Sr., and Harrower, M. : The stress tolerance test with a new projective technique utilizing both meaningful and meaningless stimuli. *Psychosom Med, 8:3,* 1946.

Grinker, R.R., Sr., and Holzman, P.: Schizophrenia in adolescence. *J Youth Adolescence, 3:*267-279, 1974.

Grinker, R.R., Sr., Korchin, S., Basowitz, H., Hamburg, O.A., Sabshin, M., Persky, H., Chevalier, J., Board, F.: A theoretical and experimental approach to problems of anxiety. *Arch Neurol Psychiatry, 76:*420, 1956.

———: Anxiety and therapy. In Masserman, J.M. and Moreno, J.L. (Eds.): *Progress in Psychotherapy.* New York, Grune, 1957, vol. 2.

Grinker, R.R., Sr., MacGregor, H., Selan, K., Klein, A., and Kohrman, J.: *Psychiatric Social Work.* New York, Basic, 1961.

Grinker, R.R., Sr., and McLean, H.: The course of a depression treated by psychotherapy and Metrazol®. *Psychosom Med, 2:*119, 1940.

Grinker, R.R., Sr., Miller, N., Sabshin, M., Nunn, R., and Nunnally, J.: *The Phenomena of Depression.* New York, Hoeber, 1961.

Grinker, R.R., Sr., Oken, D., Heath, R., Sabshin, M., and Schwartz, D.: Stress response in a group of chronic psychiatric patients. *Arch Gen Psychiatry, 3:*451, 1960.

Grinker, R.R., Sr., Persky, H., and Mirsky, I.A.: The excretion of hippuric acid in subjects with free anxiety. *J Clin Invest, 29:*110, 1950.

Grinker, R.R., Sr., Persky, H., Mirsky, I.A., and Gamm, S.: Life situations, emotions, and the excretion of hippuric acid in anxiety states. *J Clin Invest, 29:*110, 1950.

Grinker, R.R., Sr., and Robbins, F.: *Psychosomatic Case Book.* New York, Blakiston, 1954.

Grinker, R.R., Sr., Sabshin, M., Hamburg, D.A., Board, F., Basowitz, H., Korchin, S., Persky, H., and Chevalier, J.: The use of an anxiety-producing interview and its meaning to the subject. *Arch Neurol Psychiatry, 77:*406, 1957.

Grinker, R.R., Sr., and Serota, H.: Studies on corticohypothalamic relations: In the cat and man. *J Neurophysiol, 1:*579-589, 1938.

Grinker, R.R., Sr., and Spiegel, J.: *War Neurosis in North Africa: The Tunisian Campaign (January-May 1943).* New York, Josiah Macy, Jr., Foundation, 1943.

———: Narcosynthesis: A psychotherapeutic method for acute war neurosis. *Air Surgeon's Bull, 1:*1, 1944.

———: *Men Under Stress.* Philadelphia, Blakiston, 1945.

———: The returning soldier: Dissent. *Hollywood Q, 1:*321, 1946.

Grinker, R.R., Sr., and Stone, Ted: Acute toxic encephalitis in childhood. *Arch Neurol Psychiatry, 20:*244, 1928.

Grinker, R.R., Sr., and Werble, B.: Mentally healthy young men (homoclites) fourteen years later. *Arch Gen Psychiatry, 30:*701-709, 1974.

———: The second follow-up of the borderline patients. *The Borderline Patient.* New York, Aronson, 1977.

Grinker, R.R., Sr., Werble, B., and Drye, R.: *The Borderline Syndrome.*

New York, Basic, 1968.

Gruenewald, D.: A psychologist's view of the borderline syndrome. *Arch Gen Psychiatry, 23*:180-184, 1970.

Hamburg, D.A. and Adams, J.: A perspective on coping behavior. *Arch Gen Psychiatry, 17*:277, 1967.

Harrow, M., Grinker, R.R., Sr., Holzman, P.S., and Kayton, L.: Anhedonia and schizophrenia. *Am J Psychiatry, 134*:7, 1977; *Arch Gen Psychiatry, 31*:27-31, 1974; *Arch Gen Psychiatry, 34*:15-21, 1977.

Harrower, M. and Grinker, R.R., Sr.: The stress tolerance test utilizing both meaningful and meaningless stimuli. *Psychosom Med, 8*:3, 1946.

Hartmann, H.: Psychoanalysis and developmental psychology. *Essays on Ego Psychology*. London, Hogarth, 1964.

Heath, R.: Brain centers and control of behavior in man. In Nodine, J. and Mayer, J.H. (Eds.): *Psychosomatic Medicine*. Philadelphia, Lea & Febiger, 1973.

Herrick, C.J.: *George Ellet Coghill: Naturalist and Philosopher*. U of Chicago Pr, 1949.

———: *The Evolution of Human Nature*. Austin, U of Tex Pr, 1956.

Herrick, C.J. and Clarence, L.: Pioneer, Naturalist, teacher, and psychobiologist. *Trans Am Philos Soc, 45*:1-85, 1955.

Hoch, P.H. and Cattell, J.P.: The course and outcome of pseudoneurotic schizophrenia. *J Psychol, 119*:106-116, 1962.

Hoch, P.H. and Polatin, P.: Pseudoneurotic forms of schizophrenia. *Psychiatr Q, 23*:248-276, 1949.

Holland, H.: *Mental Physiology*. London, Longmans, Brown, Green and Longmans, 1952.

Holt, R.R.: In Grinker, R.R., Sr.: *Psychiatry in Broad Perspective*. New York, Behavioral Pubns, 1975, p. 95 ref.

Holzman, P.: *Psycho-analytic Research: Three Approaches to the Study of Subliminal Process*. Psychoanalytic Issues Monograph no. 30. New York, Intl Univs Pr, 1973.

———: *Psychoanalytic Research*. Psychoanalytic Issues Monograph no. 3. New York, Intl Univs Pr, 1976.

Holzman, P., Levy, D., and Proctor, L.R.: Smooth pursuit eye movements, attention, and schizophrenia. *Arch Gen Psychiatry, 33*:1414-1420, 1976.

Jackson, D.D. (Ed.): *The Etiology of Schizophrenia*. New York, Basic, 1960.

Jackson, H.: *Neurological Fragments*. Oxford U Pr, 1925.

Jacobson, E.: *Psychotic Conflict and Reality*. New York, Intl Univs Pr, 1967.

Jones, E.: *The Life and Work of Sigmund Freud, 1850-1939*. London, Basic, 1955, vols. 1-3.

Jung, C.J.: *The Undiscovered Self*. New York, Little, 1957.

Kaplan, A.: *The Conduct of Inquiry*. San Francisco, Chandler, 1964.

Katz, M., Cole, J.O., and Barton, W.E. (Eds.): *The Roles and Methodology of Classification in Psychiatry and Psychopathology.* Chevy Chase, Maryland, U.S. Dept. of Health, Education and Welfare, Public Health Service, 1968.

Kayton, L.: Clinical features of improved schizophrenics. In Gunderson, J.G. and Mosher, L.R. (Eds.): *Psychotherapy of Schizophrenia.* New York, Aronson, 1975.

Kayton, L., Beck, J., and Koh, S.: Post-psychotic state and therapeutic relationship in schizophrenic outcome. *Am J Psychiatry, 133*:11-32, 1977.

Kernberg, O.: Borderline personality organization. *J Am Psychoanal Assoc, 15*:641-685, 1967.

Kety, S.S.: Biochemical theories of schizophrenia. *Int J Psychiatry, 1*:179-200, 1967a; In Romano, J.: *The Origins of Schizophrenia.* Amsterdam, The Netherlands, Excerpta Medica Foundation, 1967b.

Kety, S.S., Rosenthal, D., Wender, P.H., and Schulsinger, F.: The types and prevalence of mental illness in the biological and adoptive families of adoptive schizophrenics. *J Psychiatr Res, 6*:345-362, 1968.

Kelin, D.F.: Psychopharmacology and the borderline patient. In Mack, J.E. (Ed.): *Borderline States in Psychiatry.* New York, Grune, 1975.

Klein, M.: *Contributions to Psychoanalysis.* London, Hogarth, 1948.

Knight, R.: *Borderline States in Psychoanalysis, Psychiatry, and Psychology.* New York, Intl Univs Pr, 1954.

Koh, S.D.: Short term memory in schizophrenic young adults. *J Nerv Ment Dis, 163*:88-101, 1976; *J Abnorm Psychol, 87*:300-313, 1978.

Kraepelin, E.: *Dementia Praecox and Paraphrenia.* Translated by R.M. Barclay. Edinburgh, E. and S. Livingstone, 1910.

———: *Clinical Psychiatry,* 7th ed. Translated by A.R. Diefendort. New York, Macmillan, 1912.

Langer, S.: Philosophical Sketches. New York, Mentor Bks, 1914.

Levinson, D.J.: The mid-life transition: A period in adult psychosocial development. *Psychiatry, 40*:99-113, 1977.

Lewin, B. and Ross, H.: *Psychoanalytic Education in the United States.* New York, Norton, 1960.

Lillie, R.S.: *General Biology and Philosophy of Organism.* U of Chicago Pr, 1945.

Lishman, W.A.: *Organic Psychiatry.* Oxford, England, Blackwell Scientific Publications, 1978.

Lipowski. A.J.: Psychosomatic medicine in the seventies: An overview. *Am J Psychiatry, 134*:233-244, 1977.

Luborsky. L., Singer, B., and Luborsky, L.: Comparative studies of psychotherapies. *Arch Gen Psychiatry, 32*:995-1021, 1975.

Mahler, M.S.: A study of the separation-individuation process and its possible application to borderline phenomenon in the psychoanalytic situations. *Psychoanal Study Child, 26*:403-424, 1971.

Mann, T.: Address, Library of Congress, 1942-1949.

Marcus, R.L.: The nature of instinct and the physical basis of libido. *Gen*

Systems, 7:133-143, 1962.

Marmor, J.: *Modern Psychoanalysis.* New York, Basic, 1968.

Meehl, P.E.: Some ruminations of the validation of clinical procedures. *Can J Psychol, 13*:102-128, 1959.

Menaker, E. and Menaker, W.: *Ego in Evolution.* New York, Grove, 1965.

Mendelson, M.: *Psychoanalytic Concepts of Depression,* 2nd ed. New York, Halsted Pr, 1974.

Menninger, K.: *The Vital Balance.* New York, Viking Pr, 1963.

Millon, G. (Ed.): *Theories of Psychopathology and Personality,* 2nd ed. Philadelphia, Saunders, 1973.

Minuchin, S.: *Families and Family Therapy.* Cambridge, Harvard U Pr, 1975.

Mirsky, I.A.: Some comments on psychosomatic medicine. The Saul Albert Memorial Lecture. *Excerpta Medica, 187*:107-125, 1968.

Mitchell, S.W.: Fifteenth anniversary address. *Transactions of the American Medico-Psychological Association,* Atlantic City, New Jersey, 1894.

Moos, R.: *Coping and Adaptation.* New York, Basic, 1974.

Mora, G.: Historical and theoretical trends in psychiatry. In Freedman, A.M., Kaplan, H.I., and Sadock, B.K. (Eds.): *Comprehensive Textbook of Psychiatry,* 2nd ed. Baltimore, Williams & Wilkins, 1975.

Mora, G. and Brand, J.L. (Eds.): *Psychiatry and Its History.* Springfield, Thomas, 1970.

Moss, D.M. III: An interview with Roy R. Grinker. *Pilgrimage, 3*:23-35, 1975.

Murphy, G.: *A Biosocial Approach to Origins and Structures.* New York, Harper Bros., 1947.

Murphy, L.B.: *The Widening World of Childhood.* New York, Basic, 1962.

Myuskonic, B.: Loneliness: An interdisciplinary approach. *Psychiatry, 40*: 113-122, 1977.

Nair, V.: Studies on the binding of drugs to plasma proteins. *Fed Proc, 23*:282, 1964.

Offer, Mahron, F., and Ostrov, E.: *The Psychological World of the Juvenile Delinquent.* New York, Basic, in press.

Offer, D. and Sabshin, M.: *Normality.* New York, Basic, 1961.

Oken, D. et al.: Relation of physiological response to affect. *Arch Gen Psychiatry, 6*:336-351, 1962.

Osler, W.: The faith that heals. In Dubos, R.J.: *The Professor, the Institute, and DNA.* New York, Rockefeller, 1976.

Perry, C. and Klerman, G.L.: The borderline patient. *Arch Gen Psychiatry, 35*:141-153, 1978.

Piers, G. and Singer, M.: *Shame and Guilt.* Springfield, Thomas, 1953.

Peterson, A.: Adolescent development from ages 16-19. In Nishpitz, J. (Ed.): *Handbook of Child Psychiatry.* New York, Basic, in press.

Popper, K.P.: *The Logic of Scientific Discovery.* London, Hogarth, 1959.

———: *Objective Knowledge.* London, Oxford U Pr, 1972.

Rado, S.: *Collected Papers.* New York, Grune, 1956 .

Rainer, J.D.: Genetics and psychiatry. In Freedman, A. and Kaplan, R. (Eds.): *Comprehensive Psychiatry.* Baltimore, Williams & Wilkins, 1973.

Rackoff, V.M., Stanas, H.C., and Kedward, H.B. (Eds.): *Psychiatric Diagnoses.* New York, Brunner-Mazel, 1977.

Roth, M.: Depressive states and their borderlands. *Compr Psychiatry, 1:* 135, 1960.

Royce, J.R.: *Psychology and the Symbol.* New York, Random, 1965.

Ruesch, J.: The infantile personality: The core problem of psychosomatic medicine. *Psychosom Med, 10:*134, 1948.

———: Psychosomatic medicine and the behavioral sciences. *Psychosom Med, 23:*277, 1961.

———: *Knowledge in Action.* New York, Aronson, 1975.

Ruesch, J. and Bateson, G.: *Communication: The Social Matrix of Psychiatry.* New York, Norton, 1951.

Ruitenbek, H. (Ed.): *Freud As We Knew Him.* Detroit, Wayne State U Pr, 1973.

Schafer, R.: *Language and Insight.* New Haven, Connecticut, Yale U Pr, 1978.

Schmale, A.H.: Relation of separation and depression. *Psychosom Med, 20:*259, 1958.

Schmideberg, M.: The borderline patient. In Arieti, S. (Ed.): *American Handbook of Psychiatry.* New York, Basic, 1969, vol. 1, pp. 398-418.

Schwab, J.S.: A response to the anti-psychiatry movement. *Psychosomatics, 18:*4, 1957.

Schwartz, D., Grinker, R.R., Sr., Harrow, M., and Holzman, P.: Six clinical features of schizophrenia. *J Nerv Ment Dis,* in press.

Schwartz, E.: Letter to Jefferson.

Scott, J.P. and Senay, E. (Eds.): *Separation and Depression.* American Association for the Advancement of Science Bulletin no. 4. Washington, D.C., AAAS, 1973.

Selye, H.: The evolution of the stress concept. *Am Sci, 61:*692-698, 1973.

———: *Stress in Health and Disease.* New York, Butterworths, 1976.

Shakow, D.: Some observations on the psychology of schizophrenia. *J Nerv Ment Dis, 153:*300-316, 1971.

Shanfield, S., Tucker, G.J., Harrow, M., and Detre, T.: The schizophrenic patient and depressive symptomatology. *J Nerv Ment Dis, 151:*203-210, 1970.

Sheldon, W.H.: Constitutional psychiatry. In Million, G. (Ed.): *Theories of Psychopathology and Personality,* 2nd ed. Philadelphia, Saunders, 1973.

Shepherd, M.: A representative psychiatrist: The career and contributions of Sir Aubrey Lewis. *Am J Psychiatry, 134:*7-14, 1977.

Spitz, R.A.: Relevance of direct infant observations. *Psychoanal Study*

Child, 5:66-75, 1950.

Spitzer, R. and Sheehy, M.: DSM III: A classification system in development. *Psychiatr Ann, 6*:102-109, 1976.

Stent, G.S.: Limits to the understanding of man. *Science, 187*:1051-1057, 1975.

Stone, A.A.: Recent mental health litigation: A critical perspective. *Am J Psychiatry, 134*:273-279, 1977.

Strauss, A., Schatzman, L., Bucher, R., Ehrlich, D., and Sabshin, M.: *Psychiatric Ideologies and Institutions.* New York, Free Pr, 1964.

Strupp, H.H.: Toward a reformulation of the psychotherapeutic influence. *Int J Psychoanal, 2*:263-365, 1973.

Summers, F. and Walsh, F.: The nature of the symbiotic bond between mother and schizophrenic. *Am J Orthopsychiatry, 47*:484-494, 1977.

Szasz, T.: *The Myth of Mental Illness.* New York, Har-Row, 1961.

———: *Schizophrenia: The Sacred Symbol of Psychiatry.* New York, Basic, 1977.

Tabachnick, N. (Ed): *Accident or Suicide?* Springfield, Thomas, 1973.

Thompson, L.: *The Secret of Culture.* New York, Random, 1969.

Torrey, E.F.: *The Death of Psychiatry.* Radnor, Pennsylvania, Chilton, 1974.

Vaillant, G.F.: The prediction of recovery in schizophrenia. *J Nerv Ment Dis, 135*:534-543, 1962.

Vale, J.R.: Role of behavior genetics in psychology. *Am Psychol, 28*:871-882, 1971.

Vick, N.: *Grinker's Neurology,* 7th ed. Springfield, Thomas, 1976.

Vieth, I.: *Hysteria: The History of a Disease.* U of Chicago Pr, 1967.

Wallerstein, R.S.: The current state of psychotherapy. *J Am Psychoanal Assoc, 14*:183-225, 1966.

Wallerstein, R.S. and Smelser, N.J.: Psychoanalysis and sociology. *Int J Psychoanal, 50*:693-716, 1969.

Walsh, F.: Concurrent grandparent death and birth of schizophrenic offspring: An intriguing ending. *Fam Process,* in press.

Watson, C.G.: Relationship of anhedonia to learning under various contingencies. *J Abnorm Psychol, 80*:43-48, 1972.

Weiss, P.: Experience and experiment in biology. *Science, 136*:468-471, 1962.

———: *The Science of Life.* Mount Kisco, New York, Futura Pub, 1973.

Werble, B.: Second follow-up of borderline patients. *Arch Gen Psychiatry, 23*:3-7, 1970.

Wheelis, A.: The vocational hazards of psychoanalysis. *Int J Psychoanal, 37*:171, 1956.

Whyte, L.L.: *The Next Development in Man.* New York, Henry Holt Co., 1948.

Williams, R.J.: *Biochemical Individuality.* New York, Wiley, 1956.

Winokur, G.: *Manic Depressive Illness.* St. Louis, Mosby, 1969.

Wolpert, E.A.: *Manic Depressive Illness as an Actual Neurosis.* New York, Intl Univs Pr, 1977.

Wortis, J.: Fragments of a Freudian analysis. *Am J Orthopsychiatry, 10:* 843-850, 1940.

Wynne, L. and Singer, M.D.: Thought disorder and family relations of schizophrenics. *Arch Gen Psychiatry, 9:*191-198, 1963.

Zilboorg, G.: *Mind, Medicine, and Man.* New York, Harcourt, Brace & Co., 1943.

Zubin, J.: On the powers of models. *J Pers, 20:*430-439, 1952.

———: Scientific models for psychopathology in the 1970's. *Semin Psychiatry, 4:*283-296, 1972.

INDEX

C

D

G

H